Phrase-book for care-givers

医師・看護師の
英語フレーズブック

Kai
SHORIN

Forward

Talking to your doctor is hard in your mother tongue. Imagine what it must be like to be sick and far from home. How do I communicate the essence of my illness to a physician whose knowledge of English is acceptable, but who cannot really understand what I am trying to say. To do the best for patients we must communicate clearly. The style of questions and caregiver responses during a taking of a medical history, for example, may elicit some unintended discomfort, or embarrassment, perhaps subconsciously. To help fill this gap Sato and Butler have created this medical phrasebook for Japanese caregivers.

It is a useful addition to what doctors and nurses can bring to their relationships with their patients. It avoids strict translations, for the nuances of good communication. This book provides a large number of common Japanese phrases, emphasizing their English equivalents over their strict English translations. In addition, it is sufficiently small in size that it can fit in your pocket. Finally, it has a thorough index for easy reference.

I would like to emphasize that these issues are not peculiar to medical care of foreigners in Japan. The problem of miscommunication, and consequent decrease in the quality of patient care and management is world-wide, and likely to become more so in the growing global community. The promotion of sensitive and non-judgmental conversations between caregivers and patients, and with attention to cultural differences is an important goal for all of us. To the extent that this little phrasebook fits this niche, one might hope that it may be a kind of model for other cultures as well.

I am pleased to recommend this phrasebook, and I look forward to learning how its implementation and use in Japan furthers the improvement of patient care.

Jeffrey M. Drazen, M.D.
Editor-in-Chief, New England Journal of Medicine
Distinguished Parker B. Francis Professor of Medicine,
Harvard Medical School

前書き
Jeffrey M. Drazen, MD の序文の和訳

　医者に話をすることは自国語でも難しい．病気になり，しかも自国から遠く離れているということがどんなことなのか，想像して欲しい．英語の知識は十分でも，患者が言おうとしている本当の意味を理解できない医師に，病気の核心を伝えることはできないだろう．患者に最善を尽くすために，私どもは明確な医師の疎通を図らなければならない．たとえば，病歴をとる際の医師の質問の仕方や医療従事者の反応は，恐らく無意識のうちに，意図しない不快感や困惑を引き出すかもしれない．このような溝を埋める一助として，著者らは日本の医療従事者のために，この臨床フレーズブックを作成した．

　この本は，医師と看護師が患者と関係を築く際の，新たな実用的ツールになるものと思う．この本は，上手に意思伝達をするのに必要なニュアンスを出すため，直訳を避けている．従って，厳密な英訳ということよりは，日英両語の該当表現に重きを置き，慣用的な日本語の言い回し（フレーズ）を多数掲載した．しかも，ポケットにピッタリ収まるよう，サイズを小さくしてある．巻末には，詳細な索引をつけて本文を参照しやすくしている．

　私は，冒頭に述べた問題が，日本における外国人の治療に特有な問題ではないことを，強調したい．誤った伝達，それによってもたらされる患者ケアと管理の質の低下は，世界規模の問題であり，社会がグローバル化し続ける中で，今後益々そうなっていく可能性がある．医療従事者と患者間の，一方的な判断をせず気配りのある，文化の違いに配慮しつつ交わされる会話の促進は，われわれすべての重要な目標である．この本が，意思伝達上のこの窪みを埋めることに寄与するとすれば，日本のみならず他文化の国々や地域にとっても，一つのモデルになる可能性を期待してもよいように思う．

　私はこのフレーズブックを推薦する．そして，日本におけるこの本の活用がどのように患者ケアの改善に役立っているかについての知らせを，楽しみにしている（訳：佐藤　忍）．

序文

　都市のみならず地方でも，英語を話す外国人患者を診察する機会が増えている．そんな中，私は，宮城県塩釜市で，冷や汗をかくことがあり，これがこのブック編纂の契機となった．そのとき私は，高校の英語教育のために来日していた英国人教師を診察した．前胸部の聴診後，背部の聴診のため"Turn your back on me, please." と言った．「背中を向ける」の訳語として，手もとの辞書から得たフレーズだった．患者は何も言わず後ろを向いてくれ，私は目的を達した．後日，共著者であるButlerから，これは，相手に不満や不服従などを表す不穏当な表現だと知らされた．失敗の理由はもちろん，私が訳語を十分吟味しなかったことにある．しかし，もし，あの辞書が，「外国人患者と日本人医療従事者間のコミュニケーションを助ける」ことに重点を置いて編集されていれば，最初に "turn around" が出てきたのではないかと思う．

　このフレーズブックは，この種の失敗がなくなることを願い「医療現場にふさわしい英語表現」を，第一のコンセプトとして作った．第二のコンセプトは，市販の多くの臨床英会話本には，索引がない．あったとしても，索引から目的のフレーズに到達するのに手間のかかることが多い．このブックでは「索引が豊富で，かつ素早くNative speakerの言い回しに到達できる」ことに重きを置いた．このため，索引ページだけで目的に到達することもあるものと思う．第三のコンセプトは，医学用語を極力使わず，「巷の日本語を巷の英語に訳す」こととした．外国人患者を妙な気持ちにさせない「良いコミュニケーション」を心掛けている多くの医療スタッフの役に立つことを願っている．

佐藤　忍

Preface

Superior medical care and patient management begins with the doctor/patient relationship. It is widely acknowledged that this is important, and that mutual respect and understanding as well as a compassionate and non-judgmental manner on the part of the physician are key ingredients of successful patient care.

Japanese physicians in clinical practice are occasionally called upon to see foreign patients, whose Japanese is inadequate for effective communication about medical issues. These individuals are often English speakers, either native or reasonably fluent in English as a second language. There are at least three difficulties in treating such patients when they visit clinics or hospitals in Japan. First, the Japanese physician often has a strong command of written English, and a large vocabulary of medical terms. However, many native or second language English speakers do not understand medical English, and this becomes a barrier to communication. Second, it is not uncommon for Japanese physicians to have less command of spoken English, and communication is sometimes hampered by this difficulty. Third, nuances and tone of phrasing are often important, especially in the initial interview and examination of patients. In particular, certain phrases may carry a negative or judgmental tone, even though that is not intended.

Our goals in preparing this phrasebook are to address, at least in part, these issues. We have been guided by the following ideas.

1. The phrasebook must be easy to use. It must be modest in length and pocket-size, and must be easy to reference desired categories of phrases.

2. It is ordered roughly as though a complete physical examination were being performed. We have collected a number of common phrases that might be used by a Japanese clinician, and have provided side-by-side a rough English equivalent. Note that these are not translations; we have tried to keep the essence of the phrases but without any kind of strict adherence to formal translation. The English phrases should be neutral and nonjudgmental in tone, and should be

limited in vocabulary to common words that are more universally understood by non-medical individuals.

3. It must have an index for easy cross-reference of terms and phrases.

With respect to the order of presentation, we follow the typical SOAP paradigm practiced by most Japanese physicians: the Subjective category includes patient symptoms and history, the Objective category includes signs found on physical examination and orders for laboratory or specialized tests, the Assessment category includes a working diagnosis, and the Plan category includes treatment plans and therapeutic interventions, medication, and follow-up. In addition, we have also added a chapter on phrases that might be most helpful to nurses, as well as a chapter on other phrases that do not fit neatly into this scheme.

To the extent that this phrasebook finds its way into the hands of practicing clinicians and nurses and helps them to overcome the ever-present language barriers that impede effective communication, thereby leading to improved medical practice and patient care, then our ultimate goals will have been fulfilled. We hope this to be the case, and welcome comments from users of this little book about their experiences with it, and how it may be improved in the future.

James P. Butler

Acknowledgements

A number of people have helped us greatly in producing this little phrasebook. We would like to especially acknowledge the help of Drs. Miki Morimoto (palliative care, currently in child care in the U.S.), Maki Shimaya (Internal Medicine, currently in Japan), Hatsuho Mamata (Radiology, currently in the U.S.), and Ms. Kimiko Sato in Japan. Whatever errors remain are entirely ours, however. We are especially and immensely grateful to Dr. Yasuharu Tokuda (Professor, Institute of Clinical Medicine, Graduate School of Comprehensive Human Sciences, University of Tsukuba) for his enthusiastic support and for introducing us to our publishers. Without the help of these individuals, this project would never have come to light.

凡例と編集方針

● 本文
- 一群の本文をグループと称し，グループの並び順に，通し番号を付けた．通し番号の下に，そのグループのキーワードを載せた．
- チーム医療における看護の重要性に鑑み，看護師が使う頻度の高いフレーズも盛り込んだ．並べ順は下記表の通り SOAP パラダイムを基本とし，S→O→A→P→Nurs→Oth の順にした．これらドメインの下に，訴え，問診，身体的検査，検査室検査，評価と説明，計画，看護過程，その他の7章を，この順に配置した．更にそれぞれの章中で，内容を大まかに，全体，頭部・顔面・頸部，胸部，背部，上肢，腹部，腰部，下肢，陰部，皮膚，その他の部位に分け，基本的にこの順に配置した．

表：本文の並べ順と章立て

(S) Subjective category
　　Chapter-1 訴え　Complaints
　　Chapter-2 問診　Interviews

(O) Objective category
　　Chapter-3 身体的検査　Physical examinations
　　Chapter-4 検査室検査　Laboratory examinations

(A) Assessment category
　　Chapter-5 評価と説明　Assessments and explanations

(P) Plan category
　　Chapter-6 計画　Plans

(Nurs) Nursing process category
　　Chapter-7 看護過程　Nursing processes

(Oth) Others category
　　Chapter-8 その他　Others

・和文本文中のxxx（類：○○○）および英文本文中のxxx (or: △△△) の意味．文脈上，○○○はxxxと，△△△はxxxと類義語であることを示す．例：「たばこも一因（類：原因の一つ）です」．医師は患者に，通常，「一因です」よりは「原因の一つです」と言う．しかしユーザーは「原因の一つです」という語句を，索引語として想起しにくい．とっさの想起という点では「一因」の方が適切という理由で，このようにした．こうすれば汎用語句をより多く掲載できる事も理由の一つである．

・英文本文中，ローマン体は医療提供側の，イタリック体は患者・家族など医療を受ける側の言葉とした．

●索引

・索引フレーズ行の先頭に，参照すべきグループを指示するため，グループ番号を付した．

・和文索引の（　）の言葉を，その索引の頭に付けてできる語句が，和文本文中の語句となる．例：「つかむ（箸で）」の場合は，テキストに「箸でつかむ」という語句があることを意味する．こうすることで，利用者は，見つけた"短い索引"からテキスト"全体における意味"を，"素早く捉える"ことができる．

・英文索引には，英文本文の"和文索引の意味を含む部分"を"切り取って"掲載した．これにより，英会話の上級者は，索引だけで目的を達する場合が多いものと思う．切り取られた英文索引が文の形をなしていても，切り取られた部分に「?」や「.」がなければ，これらの符号はつかないことになる．

・和文索引の動詞は原則として現在形とし，フレーズが命令形の場合は，表現を和らげるため「～して下さい」形式で掲載した．

・WH疑問文を含む索引は，原則的に疑問形で出した．非WH疑問文の場合は平叙文に直して出した．しかし，"any", "ever" を含む疑問文は，肯定文中では特別の意味を有するので，疑問文のまま掲載した．

著 者

James P. Butler, Ph.D.

Associate Professor Medicine,
Departments of Neurology and Medicine,
Brigham and Women's Hospital and Harvard Medical School.

Senior Lecturer in Physiology,
Molecular and Integrative Physiological Sciences Program,
Department Environmental Sciences,
Harvard School of Public Health.

医学博士 佐藤　忍

(元) 山形大学医学部第一内科助教授,
同大同学部看護学科教授

(現) 社会医療法人みゆき会みゆき会病院内科,
山形大学医学部看護学科非常勤講師

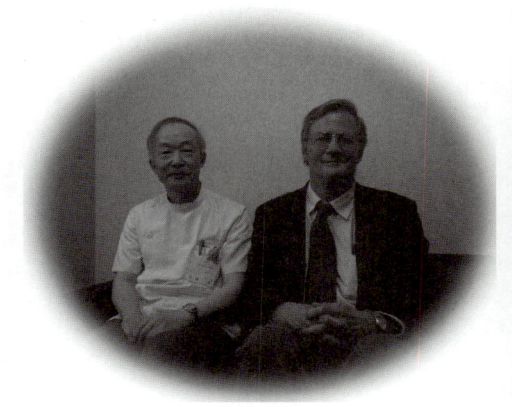

Phrase

Chapter-1 …… 訴え complaint

グループ No

1 気分
気分がぱっとしません．
I don't feel well.

2 気分
ボーッとしています．
I don't feel alert.

3 顔色
顔色が悪いです．
He looks pale.

4 気分
気持ちが落ち着きません．
I'm restless.

5 気分
元気が出ません．
I have no energy.

6 意識障害
父の意識がはっきりしないようです．
My father seems alert but a bit confused.

7 痙攣，共同偏視
父は仰向けに倒れ、手足が痙攣しました．眼は天井を向き、白眼を出していました．
My father fell down on his back. His arms and legs were cramping. His eyes were focused on the ceiling and rolled back.

8 物忘れ，聞き返す
最近、母の物忘れがひどくなり、何回も同じことを聞き返します．
Recently, my mother's forgetfulness has become worse. She asks the same things repeatedly.

9 物忘れ，昔の事，最近の事
母は、昔のことは思い出せますが、最近のことは覚えられないようです．
It seems that my mother can remember things of the past, but can't recall recent things.

10 食欲
食欲がありません．
I've lost my appetite. My appetite is poor.

11 薬物治療
最近、糖尿病の薬を飲み(類：薬物治療を)始めました．
Recently, I began taking drugs (or: medication) for diabetes.

12 低血糖
腹がすくと気分が悪くなり、冷や汗が出ます．甘い物を食べると良くなります．
I feel bad and break into a cold sweat when hungry. Eating sweet things makes me feel better.

13 全身倦怠感
どんなことをしても、疲れが抜けません．
I feel tired no matter what I do.

グループNo		
14 微熱	微熱があるようです.	*I think I have a low grade fever.*
15 顔鏡非対称	顔が少し歪んで(類：曲がって)います.	*My face feels a bit crooked.*
16 構音障害	呂律が回りません.	*I can't speak distinctly.*
17 顔面神経麻痺, 流涎	口の片側からよだれが流れます.	*I drool from one side of my mouth.*
18 疼痛,喉の奥	喉の奥が痛いです.	*My throat's sore way in the back.*
19 ドライアイ, 口内乾燥感	口が乾いて物の味がよくわかりません.眼も乾いて、チカチカする感じです.	*My mouth is dry and food seems to lose its taste. My eyes are dry and irritated, too.*
20 頭重感	頭が重いです.	*My head feels heavy.*
21 気分不良	頭がはっきりしなく、モワーッと鍋でもかぶっている感じです.	*My head's not clear. My mind's foggy and feels heavy.*
22 腫張,熱感	おでこが赤く腫れて熱をもっています.	*My forehead is red and feels hot and swollen.*
23 頭に当たる	ボールが頭に当たりました.	*A ball hit me on the head.*
24 階段踏み外し, 手すり,こぶ	階段を踏み外して頭を手すりにぶつけました.こぶができています.	*I tripped on some stairs and hit my head on the handrail. I have a bump on my head.*
25 流涙	涙眼で、涙が多いです.	*My eyes water.*
26 複視	物が二つに見えます.	*I see double.*
27 眼前霧視感	眼に霞がかかっているようで、ぼんやりしか見えません.	*My vision is blurry.*
28 黒内障	15分位の間、右眼が全く見えなくなりました.	*I went blind on the right side for 15 minutes.*
29 眼瞼浮腫, 前頚部腫脹	まぶたが腫れています.喉(類：前頚部)も腫れています.	*My eyelid is swollen. My throat is swollen, too.*

Phrase

グループNo		
30 眼内異物	眼にごみが入りました．	
	I have a speck in my eye.	
31 花粉症	毎年今頃、くしゃみが出て、眼が痒くなります．鼻がムズムズします．	
	Every year at this time, I get the sneezes, and my eyes and nose are itchy.	
32 嚥下障害	食べ物がつっかえる感じがします．	
	I have difficulty swallowing.	
33 乳房陥凹	乳のここが凹んでいるように見えます．	
	This part of my breast looks indented.	
34 乳汁漏	乳首からつゆが出てきます．	
	There's a discharge from my nipple.	
35 背部痛	身体をひねると、背中に痛みが走ります．	
	There's a sharp pain in my back when I twist.	
36 背部の重苦感	背中が重苦しい感じです．	
	I feel heaviness in my back.	
37 毛包炎、癤	背中におできができて、ズキズキ痛みます．膿んでいるように見えます．	
	I have a pimple on my back that throbs and hurts. It looks like it has pus in it.	
38 腫瘍、表在リンパ節腫脹	腋の下(脚の付け根、首)にしこりが触れます．	
	I feel a lump in my armpit (groin, neck).	
39 肩こり	肩が凝って仕方がありません．	
	My shoulder feels stiff (or: I have a stiff shoulder), and nothing seems to help.	
40 上肢運動神経麻痺	箸で食べ物をつかもうとすると、落としてしまいます．	
	I drop food from my chopsticks.	
41 手の知覚神経麻痺	手の感覚がにぶく感じます．	
	There's a dull or numb sensation in my hand.	
42 手のこわばり感	朝起きた時に手がこわばっていて、手を握る時に違和感があります．	
	My hands are stiff when I wake up in the morning, and I have a funny feeling when I make a fist.	

complaint

3

グループ No		
43 疼痛の日内変動 疼痛部位の移動	こわばり感は昼前には楽になりますが、節々が痛み、痛い所が移ります．	
	The stiffness is better by noon, but the joint soreness moves around.	
44 竹のトゲ	ささくれだった竹のとげが手に刺さりました．抜いたけど，中に残っています．	
	I got a bad bamboo splinter in my hand. I pulled it out, but there's some left.	
45 つき指	野球をしていてつき指をしました．	
	I jammed my finger playing baseball.	
46 ソ径ヘルニア	脚の付け根が膨らんでいます．横になるとひっこみ，立つと出て来るのが常でした．時に痛くなることもあります．かなり前からこの徴候はありましたが，最近は，寝てもそのままで，ひっこまなくなりました．	
	I have a bulge in my groin. It used to go away when I lay down and stick out when I stand up. Sometimes it hurts. This started a while ago, but now it's still there when I lie down.	
47 健診 大腸がん， 二次検診	年に一度の健診を受けました．便潜血検査が陽性で貧血があるため，二次検診を受けるよう，通知を受けました．	
	I had an annual health checkup. I was told to get a second medical check because the stool blood test was positive and the blood was anemic.	
48 急性腰痛症， 椎間板ヘルニア， 年のせい	腰が痛く，ぎっくり腰のようです．以前，椎間板ヘルニアになったことがあり，整形の医者から，年のせいで仕方がないと言われました．でも，何とかもっと良くならないかと思い，来ました．	
	My lower back hurts, like I strained it. I had a slipped disc before, and an orthopedic doctor said it was age related and there was nothing that could be done. But I still hope something's possible.	
49 生理痛	ひどい生理痛です．	
	I have severe cramps.	
50 歩行障害	歩くとよろめいて，右に寄って行きます．	
	I stagger and move to the right when walking.	
51 脚の疼痛	長く歩くと脚が痛くなります．	
	My legs hurt when I walk a long way.	

Phrase

52
下肢運動神経麻痺

右脚が上がりません．

I can't lift my right leg.

53
転倒，擦過傷

自転車で転んで膝と肘を擦りむきました．砂や小石がまだ残っているようです．

I fell off my bike and scratched my knees and elbows. It feels like some sand or dirt is left inside.

54
落下物，受傷

壁からブロックが落ちてきて，脚に怪我をしました．

Some bricks from a wall fell on me, and my leg got hurt.

55
足首捻挫，ハイヒール

踵の高い靴を履いていて足首をひねり，それで捻挫しました．

I twisted my ankle wearing high heels, and think I sprained it.

56
人工膝関節，セカンドオピニオン

膝が痛みます．人工関節を勧められました．セカンドオピニオンが欲しいです．

My knee hurts. An artificial knee was recommended, but I want a second opinion on that.

57
下肢運動神経麻痺

足腰に力が入りません．脚がむくみます．

My legs feel weak. My legs are swollen.

58
細かい発疹

細かい赤いぽつぽつ（類：発疹）が，全身に出ています．

I have a tiny red rash all over.

59
しみ

腕に，茶色がかったしみのようなものが出ています．

I have a kind of brownish age spot or liver spot on my arm.

60
化粧品負け

化粧品に負けました．私にはこの化粧品が合いません．

I had an allergic reaction to this cosmetic.

61
絆創膏かぶれ

絆創膏にかぶれました．

I had a funny skin reaction to the Band-Aid.

62
紫斑，あざ

腿に（脛に）紫色のあざができました．

I got a purplish bruise on my thigh (calf).

Chapter-2 …… 問診 interview

グループNo		
63 最初の言葉	どうしましたか．どこが具合が悪いですか．
	How are you doing? How are you feeling? What seems to be the trouble (or: problem)? How can I help you?
64 認知能力． 年相応． よくあること	ある程度の物忘れは、高齢者ではよくあることです．人は年をとると、しばしば物を忘れ、同じことを言うようになります．お母さんが忘れたこと、どんな時に同じことを言ったのか、例をあげて下さい．
	Some level of forgetfulness is common with age. When people grow older, they often forget things, or repeat themselves. Give me an example of something that your mother has forgotten or when she has repeated herself.
65 拍動性疼痛	その痛みはズキズキ脈打ちます（類：拍動します）か、それとも重い感じですか．
	Is the pain throbbing or dull and heavy?
66 四肢感覚障害． 嘔気	手足のしびれや吐き気はありませんか．
	Do you have numbness in your hands or legs, or any nausea?
67 四肢運動障害	手足はちゃんと動きますか、まっすぐ歩けますか．
	Are your arm and leg movements coordinated? Do you walk straight?
68 言語障害	会話（類：話をすること）が難しくないですか．いつ異常な感じに気づきましたか．
	Do you have difficulty making conversation? When did you notice this unusual feeling?
69 知覚の左右差	触った感じ、暖かさ冷たさという点で、右と左で差はありますか．
	Is there any difference in your sensations on the left or right side, in terms of touch, warmth or coolness?
70 めまい． 回転性． 浮動性． 眼前暗黒感	あなたの言うめまいは、天井や壁が回るような感じですか、船に乗っている、揺れているような感じですか、眼の前が暗くなる感じですか．
	Is your dizziness more like the ceiling or walls are rotating, like riding in a boat, or like swinging or fainting?

Phrase

71 めまい、寝返り、起立性

めまいを感じるのは寝返りする時ですか、寝ていて起き上がる時ですか.

When you feel dizzy, is it when you roll over in bed, or just when waking up?

72 立ち眩み、しゃがむ

たとえば、どんな時に立ちくらみしますか？ しゃがんでいて急に立ち上がる時ですか？

Give me an example of when you feel faint. Is it when you suddenly stand up from sitting or crouching?

73 めまい、発症後の経過

そのめまいはいつ起きましたか. めまいが起きてから今まで、程度は同じですか、軽くなっていますか.

When did the dizziness start? Is it about the same since it started, or is it better now?

74 悪寒戦慄、24時間風呂

寒気や振えはありますか. 最近、公衆浴場に行きましたか. お宅のお風呂は、24時間風呂ですか.

Do you feel chilly, and do you shiver? Have you been to a public bath recently? Does your home bath have a 24 hour system, where there is standing warm water all day long?

75 食中毒、賞味期限、いつもと違う味、悪くなる

何か悪い物を食べたという心当たりはありますか. 賞味期限が過ぎた牛乳を飲みました. 味がいつもと違う印象はありましたが、悪くなっているとは思いつきませんでした.

Do you have any idea if you ate some bad food? *I drank milk past its expiration date. I sensed an unusual taste, but I had no idea that it had gone bad.*

76 現病歴、同僚、類似症状者

家族、友人、同僚など、他のだれかに同じような症状の人はいますか.

Is there anyone else, family, friends, or coworkers who also have these symptoms?

77 食中毒、水分補給、家族内感染

水分はとっていますか. 家族のなかに、同じような症状の方はいませんか.

Did you drink something? Does your family have similar symptoms?

78 食中毒、生もの、思い当たる

生ものによる食あたりについて思い当たることはありませんか.

Do you think there's a chance of food poisoning by eating raw food (or: from raw food)?

グループNo		
79 食中毒, 生牡蠣, 食物の保管		かきを生で食べなかったですか．かきは冷蔵庫で保管していましたか．それともしばらくの間室温下に置いていましたか． *Did you have a chance to eat raw oysters? Did you keep them in a refrigerator or was there a time when you left them at room temperature?*
80 食中毒, 焼き鳥, 生焼き		食あたりと言えば，レストランで食べた焼き鳥が少し生焼けだった気がします． *Speaking of food poisoning, I remember the grilled chicken I had in a restaurant was not cooked well.*
81 インフルエンザ, 流行, 学校閉鎖		最近(類：近頃)どこかの学校が，インフルエンザの流行のため休校したと聞きました．あなたの学校はどうですか．風邪を引いている人は大勢いますか． *I recently heard that a school was closed due to an outbreak of the flu. How about your school? Are there lots of colds?*
82 学校閉鎖, 学級閉鎖		学校全体が休校したのですか．学級閉鎖をしたのですか． *Was the whole school closed, or just some classes?*
83 ワクチン接種, 健康保険		インフルエンザのワクチン(類：予防)接種は受けましたか．接種に健康保険は効きません． *Have you had a flu shot? Health insurance doesn't cover immunization shots.*
84 既往歴, ちょっと した腹痛		風邪やちょっとした腹痛以外の，一週間以上続く病気にかかったことがありますか． *Have you had any illness lasting more than a week other than a common cold or slight stomach ache?*
85 基礎代謝, 温度感覚, 平熱		汗かきですか．寒がりですか．平熱はどれ位ですか． *Do you sweat a lot? Do you often feel cold even if others do not? What is your normal body temperature?*
86 風邪の治癒日数		普段は，風邪を引いたら，何日くらいで治りますか． *When you have a cold, how long does it typically last?*
87 前医		これまで，別の医者または病院にかかっていましたか． *Have you seen another doctor or been to another hospital?*
88 前医の診断		前の医者はどんな見たて(類：診断)でしたか． *What diagnosis did your previous doctor give you?*
89 前医の処方		その医者はどんな薬を処方しましたか． *What medication did the doctor prescribe?*

Phrase

グループNo		
90 薬剤情報 提供紙	どんな薬を飲んでいますか. 薬の名前が書かれている薬局の情報提供紙(類:薬の説明書)を持っていたら, 見せて下さい. What medication are you taking? May I see the explanation forms or package insert from the pharmacy if you have them?	
91 服用薬剤	市販薬を含めて, 現在飲んでいる薬はないですか. あったら(類:もしそうなら)教えて下さい. Are you taking any drugs now, including over-the-counter drugs? If so, please tell me which ones.	interview
92 薬剤副作用	飲み薬や注射で副作用が出たことはないですか. Have you had any reactions to drugs, either oral or by injection?	
93 前立腺肥大症. 緑内障	緑内障や前立腺肥大症と言われたことはないですか. Have you ever had glaucoma or prostatic hypertrophy?	
94 家族歴. 血縁者	祖父母から子までの代の血のつながりのある人に, あなたと同じ症状の人はいますか. Are there any family members, from grandparents to children, with the same symptoms you have?	
95 既往歴. 入院する. 大きな病気	入院するような大きな病気にかかったことはありますか. 花粉症, 蕁麻疹, 風疹, はしか, 水疱瘡, 帯状疱疹はどうですか. Have you ever had a serious disease that required hospitalization? How about hay fever, hives, rubella, measles, chicken pox, or herpes zoster infections?	
96 晩酌. 休肝日	どれ位の頻度で晩酌しますか. 休肝日はありますか. How often do you drink alcohol with dinner? Are there days when you don't drink any?	
97 焼酎. 水割り	焼酎の水割りをコップ二杯飲むのですか. Do you drink two glasses of whiskey or shochu with water?	
98 食事の味付け	食事の味付けは濃いですか. 脂っこい物が好きですか. Do you like strong seasoning in food, like salt or spice? Do you like oily or fatty food?	
99 喫煙本数	タバコは一日, およそ何本吸いますか. About how many cigarettes do you smoke per day?	
100 タバコ.ふかす	タバコはふかす程度ですか, 奥まで吸い込みますか. Do you inhale tobacco smoke shallowly or deeply?	

グループNo		
101 睡眠時無呼吸、 夜間尿、 居眠り、 集中力 自動車事故	普段何時間位寝ますか．寝てから起きるまで何回目覚めますか．目覚めるたびにトイレに立ちますか．会話中に居眠りしたり、会議中に眠くなったりしますか．集中力が欠けてきたと思いますか．自動車事故を起こしたことはありますか．それは、居眠り運転が原因でしたか、それとも、ただのミスで起きたのですか．	
	How long do you sleep usually? How often do you wake up in the middle of the night? Do you go to the bathroom every time you wake up? Do you doze off when you are talking with someone? Do you become sleepy during conferences or meetings? Do you have trouble concentrating? Have you ever had a car accident? Was it because of being drowsy or was it a simple mistake?	
102 腰を抜かす、 ナルコレプシー、 むずむず脚 症候群	大笑いしたり、びっくりした時、腰を抜かしたことはありますか．寝入りばなに、たとえば無いはずの物が見えるなど、幻覚を感じたことはないですか．夢の中で金縛りになったことはありますか．眠っていて何かを蹴るような動きをしていると言われたことはありますか．	
	Have you ever frozen up when you were laughing loudly or being surprised? Have you ever had hallucinations when falling asleep, such as seeing things that aren't real? Have you ever dreamed about being paralyzed? Have you ever been told that you jerk or kick when you are asleep?	
103 コンピューター仕事	一日何時間位、仕事でコンピューターを使いますか．	
	How long during the day do you use a computer at work?	
104 仕事中の姿勢	コンピューターで仕事をする時どんな姿勢ですか．仕事中の姿勢に問題はないですか．	
	What posture do you have when working at the computer? Is there any problem with your posture?	
105 顔面神経麻痺	食べる時に口からこぼしたりしますか．	
	Do you ever drool or drop food from your mouth when eating?	

Phrase

106
咽頭痛,
嚥下痛,
口腔痛

喉のどの辺りが痛みますか. つばを飲み込む時に痛みますか. 口の中で痛いところはありますか.

Where in your throat is it sore? Does it hurt to swallow? Do you have any soreness inside your mouth?

107
洟, 痰,
後鼻漏

洟が喉の後ろを伝って落ちて, 痰になっているような感じです.

I feel like there's mucus running down the back of my throat.

108
咽頭痛,
咽後痛

喉のどこが痛みますか. 痛むのは喉の奥ですか, 前の方ですか, 首の後ろですか.

Where in the throat does it hurt? Is it in the back of your throat, or front of the throat, or all the way in the back of the neck?

109
咽頭痛,
ヒリヒリ感

喉は, 痛いというより, ヒリヒリする感じですか.

Does your throat feel like it's burning rather than simply hurting?

110
いびき,
職場の同僚,
睡眠時無呼吸,
鼻づまり

睡眠中 (類：寝ている時) に, いびきをかき, 息が止まると言われたことはありますか. たとえば職場の同僚と旅行に行った時など, 「おまえの大いびきで眠れなかった」と言われたことはありますか. それは30代でしたか. 鼻が詰まりますか.

Have you ever been told that you snore or sometimes stop breathing when you're asleep? For example, when you go on a trip with your coworker, has anyone told you that he or she couldn't sleep because of your loud snoring? Was it in your 30s? Does your nose become stuffy?

111
むち打ち症

むち打ち症など, 首を傷めたことはないですか.

Have you ever had a neck injury such as whiplash?

112
片頭痛,
眼の奥の痛み

一旦頭痛が起きるとどれ位持続しますか. 強い光, 大きな音, 階段を降りる時などに, 痛みが強くなりますか. 痛むのは頭の片側だけですか. 眼そのものあるいは眼の奥の方は痛みませんか.

How long does the pain last once it starts? Do bright lights, loud sounds, or even just walking down stairs make the pain worse? Does it hurt just on one side of your head? Do you have any pain directly in or behind your eyes?

グループNo		
113 聴力の左右差. 耳痛	耳は右左(類:両耳)で同じように聞こえますか.どちらか一方がより良く聞こえることはないですか.耳は痛いですか. Do you hear equally well in both ears, or is one better than the other? Do you have any pain in your ears?	
114 耳鳴り	耳鳴りがしますか.それはキーッという高い音ですか,ゴロゴロという低い音ですか. Do you have any ringing in your ears? Is it a high pitched squealing sound or low pitched rumble?	
115 眼痛, 痛む部位	眼がチカチカしますか.頭のどこが痛みますか Do you feel a flushness or irritation in your eyes? Where in your head does it hurt?	
116 視力, 眼鏡が合う, 複視	視力はいいですか.眼鏡をかけていますか.眼鏡は合っていますか.物が二つに見えますか. Is your eyesight good? Do you wear glasses? Is the correction proper? Do you have double vision?	
117 顔面浮腫	顔がむくんだと言われますか,あるいは顔がむくんでいると感じますか. Has anyone told you your face looks puffy? Do you think your face looks puffy?	
118 飛蚊症, 視力	眼の前で小さな虫が飛ぶような症状はありますか.眼ははっきりと見えますか. Do you have symptom such as eye floaters? Is your eyesight OK?	
119 くしゃみ, 鼻水,洟	くしゃみはよく(類:頻繁に)出ますか.洟が出ますか.鼻水はどうですか. Do you sneeze often? Do you have any nasal discharge or a runny nose?	
120 鼻づまり, 呼吸困難	鼻はつまりますか.鼻づまりで息が苦しくなりますか. Does your nose get clogged shut? Any nasal obstruction to breathing?	
121 洟の色, 鼻出血	洟の色は、黄色っぽいですか、緑がかっていますか.鼻をかむと鼻血が出ますか. What is the color of any nasal discharge? Yellowish or greenish? Do you ever get nose bleeds when you blow your nose?	

Phrase

122
洟の硬さ、粘液性、水様性

洟の硬さはどうですか. 粘液のようにドロッとしていますか, それとも水っぽいですか.

What is the consistency of any nasal discharge? Thick like mucus, or watery?

123
血縁者、気管支喘息

血縁者のだれかに喘息の人はいますか.

Do any of your blood relatives have asthma?

124
喘息気味、小中高校時代、体育をする

子供の頃に喘息気味でしたか. 小学校時代は風邪で学校をしょっちゅう休みましたか. 中学、高校時代は治療も全く必要とせず、体育もしていたのですね.

Were you asthmatic when you were a child? Were you frequently absent in elementary school due to colds? I understand you didn't require any treatment in junior high or high school, and you participated in sports.

125
喘鳴

息をする時に喘鳴が聞こえることがありますか.

Do you ever hear wheezes when you breathe?

126
咳、日内変動、空咳、湿性咳嗽

咳は、夜(夜間)も昼(日中)も、同じ強さですか. 咳で目覚めますか. 咳は空咳ですか、痰がからむ咳ですか.

Is your cough the same at night and during the day? Do you wake up coughing? Is your cough dry, or do you cough up phlegm?

127
痰の硬さ、痰の色

痰は出ますか. どんな色ですか. 硬いですか、軟らかいですか. 血が混じっていませんか.

Do you cough up phlegm (or: sputum)? What color is it? Is it thin or thick? Does it contain blood?

128
点状の血痰

痰の全体が赤いですか、ぽつんと点状に赤いのですか.

Is your phlegm uniformly reddish or spotty with tiny red spots?

129
痰の透明さ、アレルギー性、細菌感染

黄色く透明な痰はアレルギー性の病気、濁った黄色や緑色の痰は、ばい菌(類:細菌感染)による炎症の可能性が高いです. あなたの痰はどれに当てはまるか、言って下さい.

The yellowish clear phlegm may be due to an allergy. But an opaque yellowish or greenish phlegm may be due to a bacterial infection. Describe the phlegm you see.

グループNo		
130 痰の量	痰は、一日にどれ位出ますか．コップ4分の1位ですか、3分の1位ですか、それとも半分位ですか．
	How much phlegm do you produce or cough up in a day? About 1/4 (a quarter), 1/3 (a third), or 1/2 (a half) of a cup?
131 吐血． 喀血	血痰は、咳(嘔吐)と一緒に出たのですか．血痰が出る前に、トマトやチョコレートのような、赤や茶の色のついた食べ物を食べませんでしたか．血痰の中にご飯粒や、食べ物の一部は混じっていましたか．
	Did bloody sputum come out when you coughed (vomited)? Before you had bloody sputum, had you had red or brown colored food such as tomato or chocolate? Did your bloody sputum contain rice or other food pieces?
132 息切れ． 力仕事． 息切れからの回復	どんな時に息切れがしますか．じっとしていてもしますか、それとも力仕事をした時だけですか．息切れは、安静にすると、どれ位でなくなりますか．数分で元に戻りますか、何時間もかかりますか．
	When are you short of breath? Is it at rest, or is it only during physical activity? How long does your shortness of breath last after you rest? Does it take only few minutes to recover or as long as few hours?
133 自分のペースで． 他人と競争． 電柱間距離	平らな道を、だれかと競争するのではなく、あなたのペースで、休まずにどれくらい歩けますか．参考までに、電柱と電柱の間はおよそ50メートルです．
	How long can you walk at your own pace on the level without resting if you are not competing with someone? For reference, the distance between electrical poles is about 50 meters.
134 息苦しさ． 夜間覚醒	夜中に、息苦しさのために目覚めることがありますか．
	Do you wake up in the middle of the night due to shortness of breath?
135 息切れ． 日常生活動作	着替え、洗面、整容、排泄、入浴のような日常生活動作で息が切れますか．
	Are you out of breath when doing daily activities such as changing clothes, washing your face, grooming, going to the toilet, or having a bath?

Phrase

グループNo

136
上り坂，
前屈体位，
階段上がり

前かがみになる時，上り坂を上る時，階段を上がる時だけ息苦しく感じるのですか．

Do you feel out of breath only when you bend forward, climbing up a hill or stairs?

137
動悸.不整脈，
頻脈，
胸部圧迫感，
検脈

あなたの言う動悸は，脈が速くなることですか，脈が乱れることですか．動悸を感じる時，胸苦しさや胸の圧迫感はありますか．自分の脈をみることができますか．

When you say "palpitation", do you mean a fast pulse or irregular pulse? When you have palpitations, do you feel chest tightness or pressure in your chest? Can you feel your pulse?

138
動悸.労作時，
睡眠時

どんな時に動悸しがちですか，身体を動かしている時(類：労作時)ですか，安静時ですか，それとも睡眠時ですか．

When are you likely to have palpitations? Is it when you are exercising, or resting, or sleeping?

139
動悸.失神

この種の動悸は以前にも経験がありますか，それとも今回初めてですか．その時，何と診断されましたか．気を失った(類：失神した)ことはありますか．

Have you ever had this kind of palpitation before, or is this the first time? What was the diagnosis then? Have you ever blacked out?

140
痛みの強さ，
胸痛の限局性，
漠然とした

胸のどこが痛みますか．そこは，安静にしていても痛むのですか．今も痛んでいますか．痛みの強さは変わりますか．痛む場所をあなたの手で示して下さい．その場所は，指一本で示せる(類：特定できる)狭い範囲ですか，それとも，それは漠然とした範囲の痛みですか．

Where does it hurt in your chest? Does it hurt even when you are resting? Is it painful now? Does the intensity of the pain change ? Please show me the location of the pain using your hand. Can you specify the location of the pain with one finger, or is it a rather vague (or: dull) pain?

グループNo		
141 狭心痛, 疼痛間隔, ニトロール舌下, 関連痛	その痛みの間隔は段々短くなっていますか。週に何回位、痛みを感じますか。ニトロールという薬を舐めるとその痛みはより早く治まりますか。胸の痛みは他の所、たとえば、喉に通しますか。	

Is the interval between pain episodes getting shorter and shorter? How often do you have pain each week? Does the pain stop sooner if you take the medicine called "Nitorol"? Does the chest pain travel to other places such as your throat?

142
胸痛,
ゴルフスイング,
打撲,転倒,
心当たり

胸をどこかにぶっつけた、つまづいて転んだ、大きな咳をした、滅多にしないゴルフをした、など、痛みの起きた原因について、心当たりはありませんか。

Do you have any idea how this pain happened, such as hitting your chest on something, coughing violently, tripping and falling down, or even an unusual golf swing?

143
健診,
胸部写真,
要精査

健診で胸のレントゲンが引っかかったのですね。毎年健診を受けてきたが、今年初めて、精密検査を受けるように言われたのですね。

An abnormal chest x-ray was found in your medical checkup. You have a checkup every year, but this is the first time you were told to have a detailed exam.

144
嘔吐,
吐物,
腹具合

何を吐いたのですか。それはどんな色でしたか、黒っぽかったですか、黄色っぽかったですか、それとも唾のように白っぽかったですか。今は腹の具合はいいですか。

What kind of stuff did you throw up? What was the color: blackish, yellowish, or whitish like saliva? Does your stomach now feel all right?

145
胸焼け,
おくび,
胃食道逆流

胸焼けやげっぷがありますか。以前、胃食道逆流があると診断されたことはありますか。

Do you have heartburn or a burning sensation when you burp or belch? Have you been diagnosed with gastroesophageal reflux disease before?

146
腹の疼痛部位

腹のどこが痛かったですか。右上(下腹、左脇腹)が痛みましたか。腹の真ん中(臍の下)が痛みましたか。

Where did it hurt in your stomach? Did the right upper (lower, left) side of your stomach hurt? Did it hurt in the middle of your stomach (under your bellybutton)?

Phrase

グループ No		
147 疝痛, ぶり返す, 持続痛	それはキリキリと痛み、しばらくすると治まり、またぶり返しますか。それとも、波がなく続く重苦しい痛みですか。これは、これまでも、しばしばあった痛みですか。 Is it a sharp pain that goes away after a while, and comes back again? Or is it a constant, dull pain? Have you had this pain before very often?	
148 疼痛部位の 移動	最初はみぞおち辺りが痛く、その痛みが右の下腹に移ってきたのですか。 Did it hurt around the pit of your stomach at first, and then did the pain move to your lower right abdomen?	
149 受検, 胃内視鏡検査, バリウム検査	胃の検査は、バリウムでしましたか、カメラでしましたか。 Did you have a barium contrast x-ray, or a gastric camera exam for stomach checkup?	
150 普段の腹具合	腹は、普段から緩みがちですか。腹は弱い方ですか。 Do you tend to have soft stools? Do you have a weak stomach?	
151 便意,頻回	腹の落ち着きがなく、トイレに行ったすぐ後に、また行きたい感じですか。 Do you feel uncomfortable in your stomach? Do you feel like going to bathroom again soon after you go there?	
152 下部消化管 機能障害, 排ガス	下痢しがちですか、それとも便秘しがちですか。おなら(類:ガス)は出ますか。 Do you tend to have diarrhea or constipation? Do you have gas?	
153 最後の生理, 生理開始・終了, 妊娠可能性	最後の生理はいつでしたか。生理は11月16日に始まり(終わり)ました。妊娠の可能性はありますか。 When was your last period? *My period started (finished) on November 16.* Do you think you might be pregnant?	
154 生理過多, 生理不順	生理が多いですか。生理は不順でおくれがちですか。 Are your periods heavy? Is your period irregular or late?	
155 排便,便意	便通(類:排便)は毎日ありますか。便意は毎日ありますか。 Do you have a bowel movement (or: BM) every day? Do you feel like having a bowel movement every day?	

グループNo		
156 排尿痛. 排便痛	排尿する時に下腹部が痛いですか．排便する時に腹が痛みますか．	
	Does your lower abdomen hurt when you urinate? Does your stomach hurt when you have a bowel movement?	
157 タール便. 粘液便	大便(類：便)はどんな色ですか、黒くないですか、粘液のようなものは混じっていますか．	
	What color is your stool? Is it black? Does it contain what looks like a sticky fluid?	
158 頻尿. 夜間尿	頓尿についてですが、昨夜は何回トイレに起きましたか．	
	Regarding frequent urination, how often did you wake up to go to bathroom last night?	
159 頻尿. 気づく	いつ、頻尿に気づきましたか、ずっと前ですか、最近ですか．	
	When did you notice that you have frequent urination? Was it many years ago or recent?	
160 初期排尿痛. 終末期排尿痛	排尿時に痛みますか．その痛みは、排尿の始めの方で感じますか、それとも、まさに終わろうとする時ですか．	
	Does it hurt when you urinate? Do you feel pain when you start urinating or when you are about to finish?	
161 残尿感	排尿をした後でも残っているように感じる、いわゆる残尿感はありますか．	
	Do you feel a sensation called "constant urge to urinate", which means you feel like you still need to urinate even after you finish?	
162 尿の混濁. 尿の勢い	尿が濁っていませんか．尿の勢いは若い時と同じですか．	
	Is your urine cloudy or clear? Is your urine flow rate the same as when you were young?	
163 尿線の断絶	排尿の途中で、尿が途切れることはありませんか．	
	When you are urinating, do you have interrupted urine flow, or urine flow that starts and stops?	
164 排尿時の腹圧. 尿漏れ	排尿する時、腹に力を入れますか．尿漏れはありませんか	
	When you are urinating, do you have to push with your stomach? Do you have urine leakage?	

Phrase

165
グループNo
血尿，
精密検査，
放置可

初めて血尿を指摘されたのはいつですか．その時，精密検査を受けましたか．どんな検査を受けたか，詳しく教えて下さい．その結果はどうでしたか，そのまま放置していて構わないと言われましたか．

When was it first pointed out to you that you have bloody urine? Did you have a thorough examination then? Please tell me the details of the test you had. What was the result of the exam? Were you told that this is nothing to worry about?

166
いぼ痔，
坐薬

肛門からイボのような物（類：痔）が出たことはありますか．その時，坐薬を使いましたか？

Have you ever had a hemorrhoid coming out of your bottom? Have you used a suppository?

167
腓腹筋有
痛性痙攣

こむらがえりの経験がありますか．

Have you ever had a cramp in your calf?

168
水疱，
帯状疱疹

最初にどこに発疹が出ましたか．発疹は平べったかったですか，盛り上がっていましたか．それは水膨れのようでしたか．電気が走るようなピリピリする痛みがありましたか．それは痒かったですか．

Where did you have your rash first? Is it flat or raised? Does it look like blisters? Did you have a tingling pain like an electric jolt? Is your rash itchy?

Chapter-3 …… 身体的検査　physical examination

グループNo

169
顔面神経麻痺,
舌の提出,
舌下神経麻痺

ほっぺを膨らませて下さい. 舌をできるだけ前に出して下さい.
Please puff out your cheeks. Please stick out your tongue as far as possible.

170
顔面神経麻痺

微笑む、または歯を見せるように口元を横に引いて下さい.
そう、そのように.
Could you pull your lips sideways like you're smiling or showing your teeth? Yes, like that.

171
舌咽迷走神
経麻痺

口を開けて、アーッと声を出して下さい.
Open your mouth and say "Ahhh".

172
項部硬直

首の硬さ(類：項部硬直)を診ます. 枕を外します. 頭を私の手に載せて下さい.
Let me examine your neck for stiffness. I'm going to remove the pillow. Place your head on my hand.

173
眼筋麻痺

もう少し、あごを引いて下さい. 私の指先を、顔を動かさないで眼で追って下さい.
Could you please tuck in your chin a little? Follow my finger with your eyes, without moving your head.

174
眼球運動,
対面検査

まっすぐ、遠くの方を見て下さい. 私の方にまっすぐ向いて下さい.
Please look straight ahead. Now look straight at me.

175
輻輳反射

私の指先を、眼をそらさないで、ジーッと見ていて下さい.
自分の鼻先を見つめて下さい.
Please focus on my fingertip. Can you focus on your nose?

176
対光反射,
瞳孔サイズ

今から、対光反射と瞳の大きさを診ます.
Now I'm going to examine your light reflexes and the size of your pupils.

177
眼輪筋麻痺,
顔面神経麻痺

両方の眼をしっかり閉じたままでいて下さい. 鼻の孔を膨らませて下さい.
Keep your eyes closed tightly. Flare your nostrils.

Phrase

178
呼吸音聴診、深呼吸

今から胸の音を聴きます。息を吸ったり吐いたりして下さい。もう少し速くして(類：呼吸して)下さい。深呼吸をして下さい。はい、結構です。音はきれいです。全く(あまり)心配いりません。

Now I'd like to listen to your breathing. Breathe in slowly … Breathe out slowly …. Now breathe a little faster. Take a deep breath in. Good. Your breath sounds are clear, and there's nothing to worry about (Things are probably o.k.).

179
咳払い、咳嗽後ラ音

静かに息をして下さい。咳払いを二回して下さい。

Please breathe quietly. Please clear your throat twice.

180
肋間腔開大

右腕をず～っと上に、耳にくっつくまで上げ、胸の右側を突き出して下さい。

Raise your right arm all the way up until it touches your ear, and push the right side of your chest out.

181
強制呼気時聴診

できるだけ大きく息を吸い、もう吸えないとなったら、その息を、できるだけ速く吐いて下さい。

Take a deep breath in, as far as you can go. When you can't get any more air in, blow out as fast as possible.

182
脱衣

上半身を脱いで、このタオルをかけて下さい。

Please take off your top and cover yourself with this towel.

183
胸痛

胸を押します。痛い時は言って下さい。こうすると痛いですか。

I will push on your chest, so please let me know when it hurts. Does it hurt if I do this?

184
背部打聴診体位、猫背

両腕を前で交叉させ、首を前に曲げて下さい。猫背になって下さい。

Cross your arms in front of you, and tuck your chin to your chest. Please curl up into a ball.

185
打聴診体位変換

後ろを向いて下さい。背中を診察します。前向きに戻って(類：私の方を向いて)下さい。

Please turn around so I can examine your back. Now turn around and face me again.

グループ No		
186 上肢腱反射	背筋を伸ばしてかけ、腕の力を抜いて楽にして下さい．両手を膝に載せて下さい．	
	Please sit up straight, and let your arms relax. Put both hands on your knees.	
187 上肢バレー徴候	両手の手のひらを上にして、まっすぐ前に腕を伸ばして下さい．眼を閉じて10秒間そのままでいて下さい．	
	Turn your palms up and extend your arms straight ahead. Can you do this for 10 seconds with your eyes closed?	
188 手回内回外検査	両手を、このように、ギンギンギラギラするように、回して下さい．	
	Can you twirl your hands around like this?	
189 指鼻試験	人差し指を出して、腕を横に出して下さい．その指先で、自分の鼻先に触って下さい．今度は眼を閉じて、同じことをして下さい．	
	Extend your arm to one side, pointing with your first finger. Now touch your nose with your fingertip. This time, close your eyes and do the same thing.	
190 Allen試験	今から、後に立って、ある徴候を検査します．手を貸して下さい．後ろから脈をみます．腕を曲げて下さい．顔を左に向けて下さい．手がしびれますか．手から血の気が少なくなったように見えます．	
	Now I'll check some signs, standing behind you. Please give me your hand and I'll check your pulse from behind. Now flex your arm. Turn your head to the left. Is there any numbness in your hand? It looks as if there's less circulation in your hand.	
191 腹部触診・打聴診	ベッドに寝て下さい．腹を診ます．腹の力を抜いて楽にして下さい．	
	Lie back on the bed while I check your abdomen. Please relax your abdomen (or: stomach).	
192 腹部圧痛	押されて痛かったら教えて下さい．ここが痛みますか．	
	Tell me if it hurts when I press down. Does this hurt?	
193 反跳痛	手で押す時と手を離す時、どっちが痛いですか．	
	Does it hurt more when I press down or when I let up?	
194 肝脾触知	腹を膨らませて下さい．今度はへこませて下さい．	
	Push your stomach out. Now suck it in.	
195 肋骨脊椎角叩打痛	今から軽く叩きます．叩かれて痛かったら言って下さい．右と左で痛みに違い（類：左右差）はありますか．	
	I'm going to tap you lightly, and tell me if it hurts. Is there any difference in pain on the left or right side?	

Phrase

196
直腸指診

おしりを指で診察します。おしりに指を入れます。ベッドに、壁に向って横向きに寝て下さい。看護師が下着を下げます。両膝を両手で抱え、腹の方に持ち上げて下さい。すぐに終わります。はい、終わりました。指の届く範囲には何も異常を認めません。

Let me examine your anus using my finger. I will insert my finger into your anus. Please lie down on your side facing the wall. A nurse will take off your underwear. Please hold your knees with both hands and move them closer to your stomach. I will finish soon. Now it's done. I didn't recognize any abnormal area within the reach of my finger.

197
膝蓋腱反射

ベッドに腰をかけて、両脚を下げて下さい。両手をこのように組んで下さい。私がイチ、ニ、サン、ハイ、と号令をかけたら組んだ手を両側に引っ張って下さい。

Please sit up on the bed and let your legs hang down. Hold both hands like this. Then pull on them when I say "One, two, three, go".

198
アキレス腱反射

アキレス腱反射をみます。間仕切りに向き、上半身を起こし、ベッドに両膝をついて下さい。手を間仕切りに付けて身体を支えて下さい。

Let me check your Achilles tendon reflex. Put both knees on the bed facing the partition, with your upper body upright. Support your body touching the partition with both hands.

199
つま先立ち、踵立ち

両足の踵で立って下さい。次はつま先で立って下さい。

Stand on your heels, then stand on your toes.

200
ロンベルグ試験

左右の踵とつま先をくっつけて、立って下さい。

Now stand with heels and toes touching each other.

201
マン試験、片足立ち試験

片方の足をもう片方の後ろに置き、後ろ足のつま先を前足の踵につけて、立てますか? 片足で立ってみて下さい。先ず右足で。はい下ろして下さい。今度は左足で。

Can you stand with one foot behind the other, with the toes of the back foot touching the heel of the front one? Try to stand on one foot. First on your right foot. Ok, good. Now try your left foot.

グループNo		
202 踵膝試験	仰向けに寝て下さい．片方の脚を上げ，その踵を反対側の脚の膝に載せて下さい．その後，踵を足首まで，なぞり下ろして下さい．	
	Now just lie down on your back. Lift up one leg and place your heel on the other leg's knee. Now slide your heel down to the ankle.	
203 膝蓋腱反射	両膝を立てて，そのままでいて下さい．	
	Please raise your knees up and hold still.	
204 下肢の交叉	仰向けに戻り，膝を立てて，それを交叉させて重ねて下さい．力を抜いて下さい．	
	Turn back over and lie on your back. Pull your knees up, cross one over the other, and relax.	
205 振動覚	この音叉を踝に当てます．振えを感じますか？ 振えを感じなくなったら，知らせて下さい．	
	I will place a tuning fork on your ankle. Can you sense the vibration? Tell me when you cannot sense the vibration any more.	
206 ラゼーグ徴候	私がこうやって脚を上げると，腿の後ろが突っ張ったり，痛んだりしますか．	
	When I lift your leg like this, does the back of your thigh hurt or feel tense?	
207 下肢バレー徴候	ぐるっと回って腹這いになって下さい．脚を軽く，これ位曲げ，そのままでいて下さい．	
	Turn back over on your stomach (or: Please turn over and lie on your stomach). Bend your legs slightly like this and hold still.	
208 口内炎， 皮膚粘膜診	唇の内側に口内炎が起きています．口以外のどこかに，たとえば陰部や皮膚に，痛みや発疹(類：湿疹)はありますか．	
	You have a mouth ulcer inside your lip. Do you have pain or a rash elsewhere other than your mouth such as your pubic area or skin?	
209 腹壁視診， 手術痕	ここに5センチ位の傷痕がありますが，何の手術の痕ですか．	
	I see you have a 5 cm scar here. What kind of surgery was that for?	

Phrase

Chapter-4 …… 検査室検査 laboratory examination

グループNo		
210 腫瘍マーカー， 脂質， 肝機能	その血液で腫瘍マーカーと脂肪と肝機能を調べます． We will examine the blood for tumor markers, lipids and liver function.	
211 空腹時血液 検査	この次は，診察の前に，空腹時血液検査をします．受診当日の朝は，何も食べないで，おいで下さい．しかし，いつも飲んでいる薬は，水で飲んで来て(類：続けて)下さい． Next time, we'll need to take a fasting blood sample before you see the doctor. This means you should not eat anything beginning the morning of your visit. But you should continue taking your usual medicines with water.	
212 X線写真の 特性， 技師の条件 設定	レントゲン写真は技師の条件設定次第で違って見えることがあります．従って，今日の写真に異常影が見えないこともあり得ます． X-ray images can look different depending on the machine settings. Thus it is possible that we don't see any abnormal shadows in today's x-ray.	
213 睡眠モニター， 検査技師， 家族同伴， 説明時間	器機は弁当箱位の大きさで，身体に付けるセンサーは3つです．一つは呼吸センサーで，鼻の下にテープで貼り付けます．一つは血液中の酸素の量を測るセンサーで，指にはめます．最後は小さな「喉マイクロホン」で，喉仏の辺りに貼り付けます．センサーの付け方は検査技師が説明します．20〜30分かかります．説明の間，お家の方が同席するのがいいです． The machine is the size of a bento-box. There are three sensors attached to your body. One is for your mouth and nose to record your breathing, and it will be attached under your nose with tape. The second sensor is for measuring the oxygen level in the blood. You will wear that sensor on your finger. The last sensor is a small throat microphone and will be attached around your Adam's apple. A laboratory technician will explain how to attach the sensors, and the explanation will be 20-30 minutes. It would be helpful if a family member could be with you during the explanation.	

グループNo		
214 心電図, 胸部単純写真, 結果待ち時間	心電図をとります. 胸のX線写真を撮ります. 写真は20分もあればできます.	
	I will take an electrocardiogram (ECG). I will take a chest x-ray. The x-ray will be ready within twenty minutes.	
215 24時間心電図, 日常生活	お風呂やシャワー以外のことは、いつも通りして結構です. くれぐれも、いつも通りの生活(類:日常生活)をして下さい. そうしないと、結果の解釈ができなくなります.	
	You can perform all your normal daily activities except that you cannot take a bath or shower. Please make sure that you keep to your daily routine, otherwise we cannot interpret the results.	
216 胸部単純写真, 撮影体位, 見落とし	普通の写真では、一枚の写真に色々なものが重なって見えます. ほんのわずかな撮影体位の変化が異常陰影を見失う(類:見落とす)ことにつながります.	
	In one conventional image, we will see many different organs, all overlapped. Even the slightest change of position in taking x-rays can lead to missing of abnormal shadows.	
217 蓄痰	3日間痰を溜めて下さい. 溜めたら早めに病院にお持ち下さい.	
	Please collect your sputum for three days. Please bring the sputum in once you've finished.	
218 痰採取法	唾では診断できません. 胸の奥から痰を出すようにして下さい.	
	Saliva can't be used for the diagnosis, so please try to cough up the sputum from your lung.	
219 結核菌 痰塗抹検査, 培養検査	痰を容器に入れて下さい. それを二通りの方法で調べます. 一つは塗沫検査と言い、すぐに結果が分かります. もう一つは培養検査と言い、最長で8週間かかります.	
	Please put the sputum in the container. We will examine the sputum in two ways. One way is called smear examination. We will know the result soon. Another is called culture, and it will take 8 weeks at most.	

Phrase

グループNo
220
気管支鏡,
咽頭喉頭麻酔,
詳しい説明

気管支鏡は、胃カメラよりずっと細く、太さは鉛筆と同じ位です。まず、咳と吐き気を抑えるために、喉に麻酔をします。詳しいこと(類:説明)は、説明書に書かれているので、後で注意深く読んで下さい。その上でこの検査を受けるか決めて下さい。

A bronchoscope is much thinner than a gastric camera. Its diameter is about the same as a pencil. First, we will give you an anesthetic in your throat in order to prevent coughing and gagging. Detailed explanations are in the booklet, so please read them carefully later. Then you can decide whether you want to have a bronchoscopic exam or not.

221
早朝尿,
尿検査

この次に来る時、朝起きて最初の尿を持って来て下さい。そのための容器を渡します。

When you come next time, please bring your first urine sample after you wake up. I will give you the container for that.

Chapter-5 …… 評価と説明　assessment and explanation

グループNo

222
肥満,減量

標準に比べて肥っています．これ以上肥ると，膝の関節を含めて全身に問題が起きます．5キロ程度減量しましょう．

You are overweight compared with normal. If you gain more weight, you will encounter more problems throughout your body including knee joints. You should lose roughly 5 kg.

223
やせ,偏食

痩せていますね．半年でどれ位痩せましたか．食べ物に好き嫌いがありますか．

You look slim. How much weight did you lose over the past 6 months? Are you particular about foods?

224
不眠,
中途覚醒,
咳止め,
痒み止め

寝つきはいいが，夜間途中で目覚めるために日中寝不足なのでしたら，睡眠薬がいいです．痒みや咳のために良く眠れない(類：不眠な)のであれば，咳止めや痒み止めがいいです．

If you feel tired during the day, because of waking up often during the night, even though you may fall asleep quickly, I recommend some medicine for insomnia. If you wake up due to cough or itchiness, you need some cough medicine or anti-itch medicine.

225
心配事,
不安な時,
頻脈,
安定剤

何か心配事がある時，不安な時は，頻脈になり(類：脈が増え)ます．その場合は，安定剤を飲むと，気持ちが落ち着き(類：効き)，脈も落ち着くことがあります．

When you're worried or anxious, your heart rate can go up. In that case, some antidepressants can help, and bring your pulse rate down.

226
気になる,
心配

うんと気になるよう(類：心配)でしたら，薬を飲むことを勧めます．

If you're really worried, I can recommend some medicine.

227
心配無要

現時点では，心配するような所見は何もありません．

At this point there's nothing to worry about.

228
めまい,
専門科,
耳鼻科医

めまいは耳鼻科(類：耳鼻科医)が専門です．耳鼻科に紹介状を書きますので行って下さい．

You should see an ENT (ear, nose, throat) doctor, because one of their specialties is in treating dizziness. I'll give you a referral.

Phrase

グループNo

229
血液生化学, X線写真, 穏やか

血液生化学検査の結果、カリウムが少ないです。レントゲン写真の所見の割には、血液検査の所見が穏やかです。

Your blood chemistry suggests that potassium is low. The x-ray findings are of some concern, but the blood test shows relatively mild abnormality.

230
空腹時及び随時血糖値, 経口ブドウ糖負荷試験

糖尿病は、空腹時の血糖、口から飲んだブドウ糖に対する血糖値の上がり方、あるいは空腹でなくとも、受診した時点で(類:随時に)測った血糖で診断します。

Diabetes is diagnosed based on a fasting blood sugar exam, and on the response to an oral glucose drink. We may also take a measurement at the time of your visit even without fasting.

231
細胞診, 組織診

これは感染症か腫瘍か、判断がつきません。最終診断には、細胞や組織の検査が必要です。

We can't determine if this is an infection or a tumor. An exam of cells or tissue will be needed to make a final diagnosis.

232
睡眠時無呼吸器機の貸し出し

睡眠時無呼吸の疑いがあります。診断のために、自宅でできる簡単な検査があります。そのための器機は貸し出しします。

There is a possibility that you have sleep apnea. To check this, there is a simple, easy exam you can do at home. I will lend you a machine for that.

233
風邪, 持病

私は、あなたは風邪を引いただけだと思います。他に持病がなければ、安静だけで治ります。

I suspect you just have a common cold. If you don't have other chronic diseases, simply resting is enough to get well.

234
特効薬, 頓服の鎮痛剤

インフルエンザには特効薬があります。これと違って、風邪などのウィルスを退治する特効薬はありません。身体を休めて、打ち勝つ力を強くするのが治療の基本です。頭痛がひどければ頓服の鎮痛剤を飲んで下さい。

For the flu, we do have special medicine. But unlike this, we have no medicine to kill viruses such as the common cold. Treatment is basically rest, and building up your strength. If your headache is bad, you can take a painkiller as needed.

グループNo		
235 即効薬． 即効療法	たとえ旅行に行くにしても、速く治す治療法や即効薬を処方してくれという申し出は、無理です．
	Even though you may be going on a trip, there is no quick cure or medicine that I can prescribe.
236 インフルエンザ予防． 潜伏期． 手洗い． うがい	インフルエンザは、数日間の潜伏期を経て、発症します．予防には、うがい、手洗い、十分身体を休める（類：休養する）ことが大切です．
	Flu develops over a few days incubation period. In order to prevent flu, gargling, washing hands, and getting enough rest will be important.
237 筋力の衰え． 呼吸リハビリ． 役に立つ運動． 膝の屈伸	患者は、しばしば息切れを感じると、日常生活での動きを少なくしがちです．すると、足腰の筋力の衰えが引き起こされます．簡単で役に立つ（類：リハビリになる）運動があります．たとえば、腰の高さの棒につかまって、膝の曲げ伸ばしをする、椅子にかけていながら脚を上げ下げするなどです．
	If you're often short of breath, you tend to be inactive, which in turn leads to muscle weakness in your legs and lower body. There are some simple exercises that will help. For example, you can hold on to a bar at hip level and squat down and up, or move your legs up and down while sitting.
238 歯周病． 歯槽膿漏	歯磨き中や歯茎を強く吸った後に血が出る（類：出血する）とのことから、歯周炎や歯槽膿漏による出血が疑われます．タバコも一因（類：原因の一つ）です．ですから（類：だから）止めましょう（類：禁煙しましょう）．
	You said your gums bleed when you brush your teeth or suck strongly. This is likely either gum disease or perhaps an abscess. Smoking may contribute to this, so you should quit smoking as well.
239 扁桃腺周囲膿瘍． 抗生剤	扁桃腺の炎症（感染）が周囲に及んでいます．喉の所見から膿瘍の可能性があります．強力な抗生剤が必要です．
	The inflammation (infection) in your tonsil is affecting the surrounding tissue. From the appearance of your throat, an abscess is possible, so you'll definitely need an antibiotic.

Phrase

240
亜急性甲状腺炎, 副腎皮質ホルモン

甲状腺に圧痛があります. 炎症が治るにつれて痛みも軽くなります. 一時的に甲状腺ホルモンが過剰になっています. 痛みを和らげ, ホルモンを正常に戻すために, 副腎皮質ホルモンを処方します. 良性の病気ですから心配はいりません.

You have thyroid tenderness, which will get better as inflammation goes down. You temporarily have excessive thyroid hormone in your blood. I'll prescribe a steroid to ease your pain and to bring it back to normal. This condition is benign, so you don't have to worry.

241
脳出血, 悪いもの, 筋収縮性頭痛

脳出血など, 頭の中に悪いものがあるように見えません. 首の周囲の筋肉の, 過度の緊張(類:収縮)による痛みのようです. 筋収縮性頭痛には, ラジオ体操も結構有効です.

It seems there's nothing wrong in your brain, such as bleeding. I suspect your headache is due to a stiff neck and excessive muscle strain around your neck. "Rajio taiso", or radio exercise, may be helpful for tension headache.

242
MR画像処理, 早期の脳梗塞, 描出

特殊な方法で処理したMR画像では, 起きて数時間後に, 脳梗塞の影響を見ることができます. このMR血管画像では, 梗塞の領域を養う血管が見えません(類:描出されません).

In an MR image processed in a special way, we can see the effects of a stroke several hours after it developed. In this MR angiogram image, blood vessels feeding a stroke area are not visible.

243
片頭痛, 痛みを予防・和らげる薬

片頭痛は, 若い女性に多いです(類:よくみられます). 頭痛を予防すると, 起きた頭痛を和らげる薬があります.

Migraine headache is common among young women. We have two medicines, one to prevent and one to ease the pain.

244
舌下錠の用法

ニトロールは舌下錠です. 噛んだり飲み込んだりしないで, 舌の下に置いて, 自然に溶かして下さい.

Note that Nitorol is a sublingual tablet. You should place it under your tongue and let it dissolve. Don't chew it or swallow it directly.

グループ No		
245 異常呼吸音	息を吸う(吐く)時に異常な呼吸音が聞こえます. I hear a possibly abnormal sound when you inhale (exhale).	
246 心雑音. 心臓弁. 超音波検査	心臓に雑音(類:心雑音)が聞こえます.心臓の弁に問題があるようです.超音波検査をすれば,診断に役立ちます. I hear a heart murmur, suggesting a problem with the heart valves. An ultrasound examination will help with diagnosis.	
247 血管造影. 大動脈解離	造影剤を使って胸部と大きな血管の検査をしました.大動脈が心臓から出た(類:枝分かれした)直後の部分,上行大動脈に解離という所見があります.解離とは動脈の壁と壁の間が剥がれることです.恐らく解離が,胸痛の原因と判断します. We have completed the chest examination, including visualizing the aorta with a contrast agent. There is a finding called "Dissection" in the ascending portion of the aorta, which is right after it branches out from the heart. This means that the three layers of the arterial wall start to peel apart, and this is the likely cause of your chest pain.	
248 心筋梗塞. 労作性狭心症. 24時間心電図	心筋梗塞らしくはありません.労作性狭心症の疑いが否定できません.小さな心電図記録器を身体につけて,24時間記録することをお勧めします. It is not likely that you had a myocardial infarction or heart attack. We cannot rule out angina on effort. We recommend that you wear a small monitor that will record your ECG over 24 hours.	
249 CT 画像. 乳頭レベル. 輪切り像. 肺炎	このCT写真は,乳首のレベルでの輪切り像です.こっちが腹側です.この部分は他より白く見えます.このスジ状の黒い影は気管支です.気管支が中に見える影は,良性の疾患によく見られます(類:多いです).従って,肺炎の疑いが濃い(類:強い)です. This CT picture shows the cross-section at the level of the nipple. This is the abdominal side. This area looks whiter than other area. This black streak is a bronchial tube or airway. The shadow with bronchial tubes seen inside is common with benign diseases. Thus, we strongly suspect pneumonia.	

Phrase

グループNo

250
石灰化陰影

この白っぽい領域に、ひと際白い、肋骨と同じくらい白い影があります。これを石灰化陰影と言います。

There is a markedly white shadow in this whitish area. This shadow is as white as ribs. This is called a calcification shadow.

251
胸膜に接した陰影

この陰影は胸膜に接しています。胸膜を下にした台形のような形です。

This shadow is tangent to the pleura. The shape is trapezoidal, based on the pleura.

252
境界明瞭,
血管影収束,
棘形成,
空洞

この影は陰影の濃さが均一です。境界ははっきりしています(類:明瞭です)。ウニのとげのように見えるものがあります。この陰影に向かってまわりの血管が引っ張られているように見えます。内部(類:中)に空洞も見えます。

This shadow looks pretty uniform, and its edges are sharply defined. There are some structures which look like sea urchin spines. It looks like the vessels around this shadow are pulled towards it. We can also see the cavity inside.

253
胸膜と陰影のなす角度,
発育方向

胸膜とこの陰影のなす角度は90度より小さい(大きい)、鋭角(鈍角)です。これは、異常陰影が肺の方から胸膜に向かって発育したことを意味します。

The angle between this abnormal shadow and the pleural membranes is smaller (bigger) than 90 degrees, an acute (obtuse) angle. This means the abnormal shadow grows from the lung towards the pleura.

254
否定する,
痰の結核菌

陰影から結核を否定できません。痰に結核菌がいるかどうかを見る検査をしましょう。

We can't rule out tuberculosis from the shadow. Let me examine your sputum to see whether there is a tuberculosis organism.

255
心不全症候,
起座呼吸

心臓が弱っています。寝ている状態(類:臥位)から起きる(類:起座位になる)と息苦しさが軽くなる(類:改善する)症状は、その証拠の一つです(類:それを示しています)。

You have some heart weakness, as indicated by the fact that your shortness of breath improves when going from lying down to sitting up.

グループNo		
256 労作時息切れ 大丈夫, 症状の軽減	肺の病気になると、しばしば痰が出ます。このため、特に労作時などに、息切れを感じることがあります。しかしあまり心配しないで大丈夫です。あなたの症状を軽くすることはできますので.	
	Lung diseases sometimes produce sputum, which can make you short of breath, especially when exercising. But don't worry too much. We can lighten your symptoms.	
257 発作性心房細動, 血の塊, 脳梗塞	発作性の心房細動が起きています。血の塊が剥がれ、血管に詰まり、脳梗塞を起こすことがあるので、危険です。	
	You have paroxysmal atrial fibrillation. This is dangerous because of potential breaking loose of clots, blocking the vessels and causing a stroke.	
258 虫垂炎, 診断がつかない, 造影CT	虫垂炎の疑いがあるので、血液検査と腹の超音波検査をします。それでも診断がつかない時は、造影CT検査が必要です。	
	There is a possibility that you have appendicitis. Let me do a blood test and abdominal ultrasound. If we are still not sure of the diagnosis, we'll need to do a contrast CT.	
259 骨盤部CT画像, 脂肪組織の炎症像, 緊急手術	これは骨盤部のCTです。白くリング状に見えるのが虫垂の断面で、太さはおよそ1センチです。虫垂周囲の脂肪組織が、皮下脂肪と比べて、より白っぽく、もやもやと見えます。緊急の手術が必要です.	
	This is a pelvic CT. A white shadow that looks like a ring is the section of your appendix. It's one centimeter thick. The surrounding fat tissue looks more whitish and wispy as compared with subcutaneous fat. You are in urgent need of an operation.	
260 大腸憩室炎	右の下腹が痛んで熱が出る他の病気に大腸の憩室炎があります。この病気は、大腸の壁の凹みの炎症で引き起こされます.	
	One of the other diseases with fever and right-side lower stomach pain is colon diverticulitis. This disease is caused by inflammation of a small pit-like structure in the colon.	
261 胃ポリープ, 生検, 外来で可能, 入院不要	胃にポリープがあります。組織診断をする必要があります。組織検査は外来でできます。入院する必要はありません。	
	You have a polyp in the stomach, which requires a tissue diagnosis. You will not need to be admitted to the hospital. The tissue biopsy can be done in the out-patient clinic.	

Phrase

262
悪性の嚢胞性陰影は、中が凸凹に見えたり、仕切られていたり、急に大きくなったりします。

悪性嚢胞性陰影 中が凸凹

The malignant cystic shadow looks irregular inside, being partitioned or divided, or grows rapidly.

263
超音波検査で、胆嚢に石が見つかりました。定期的に追跡する必要があります。

胆嚢結石 定期的追跡

A stone has been discovered in your gall bladder by ultrasound. This should be followed up regularly.

264
石に関しては、胆嚢炎を起こしたり、胆管に落ち込んで管を詰まらせない限り、手術で摘出しないのが普通です。

胆石の手術適応 胆嚢炎 胆管閉塞

Regarding the stone, usually we don't operate to take it out unless it causes cholecystitis or falls into biliary duct and stops it up.

265
悪いものを早く体の外に出すのが望ましいです。そのため、下痢止めを使いません。整腸剤が効きます。一日3回規則的に飲む整腸剤と、頓服の痛み止めを処方します。

急性胃腸炎 整腸剤 止痢剤 頓服

Sometimes it's best to let bad things leave the body naturally, and not to take anti-diarrheal medicines. Perhaps a pro-biotic will help. I'll prescribe one for you to be taken regularly three times per day and a painkiller to be taken as needed.

266
腸閉塞です。入院して、しばらく絶食し、治療する必要があります。管でガスを抜きます。大丈夫、点滴で栄養分は入れます。

腸閉塞 絶食 点滴栄養補給

You have a bowel obstruction, which will require hospitalization. You won't be able to eat or drink for a while. But don't worry, we'll give you nutrition by i.v., and relieve your gas with a tube.

267
膀胱炎です。排尿を長時間我慢しないで下さい。尿は膀胱の中のばい菌を洗い流します。

膀胱炎 排尿を我慢 洗い流す

You have a urinary bladder infection, so please don't hold back or wait too long to urinate. The urine will wash out the bacteria.

グループNo		
268 尿路結石. ニボー. 糞塊. 浣腸. 効く	これは腹のレントゲン写真です. 腎臓や尿管の石を示唆する所見も, 閉塞した腸に液体が溜まっている所見もありません. しかし, 大量の糞塊(類:便)が大腸に溜まっています. 腹痛の原因は便秘のようです. 浣腸が効くと思います.	
	This is an abdominal x-ray image. There is no sign suggesting kidney stones, nor accumulation of fluid in the obstructed bowel. However, there appears to be excessive fecal material (or: stool) in the colon. Constipation may then be a cause of your stomach pain. I suggest an enema will help.	
269 尿沈渣. 顕微鏡的尿検査. 血尿	今日の尿の顕微鏡検査では(類:に拠れば), 一視野に4個以下の赤血球しか, 認めません. これは病的とは見なさない程度の血尿です.	
	According to today's microscopic examination, there were less than 4 red blood cells in one microscopic field. This means we don't think this is caused by disease.	
270 起立性蛋白尿. 起床直後の尿	活動すると, 蛋白尿が出る人がいます. その場合は, 起床直後の尿は正常なことが多いです.	
	Some people have protein in their urine after exercise. In that case, most of them have normal urine right after they wake up.	
271 休診時の当座・事後対応	かかりつけの皮膚科で診てもらうのがいいです. 今日は皮膚科が休みです. とりあえず, 痒み止めを処方します. 明日, 必ず皮膚科を受診して下さい.	
	You should go see your dermatologist, but since that department is not open today, I'll prescribe some anti-itch medicine for now. Make sure you go see a dermatologist tomorrow.	

Phrase

Chapter-6 …… 計画 plan

グループNo

272
有熱時治療.
飲食指示.
解熱剤

熱のある時は多目の水分を摂り、消化のいい物を食べて下さい。摂氏38度以上の熱がある時は、熱さまし(類：解熱剤)を飲んで下さい。

If you get a fever, be sure to drink lots of fluids and eat bland food. When you have temperature greater than 38 degrees Centigrade, take a fever reducing medicine.

273
インフルエンザの場合.
学校復帰

インフルエンザの場合は、解熱後(類：熱が下がってから)二日経てば学校に行ってもいいです。

With flu, 2 days after the fever goes away, you can return to school.

274
症状悪化・
持続・
ぶり返し.
再受診勧奨

症状が続く、悪くなる、あるいは良くなってからぶり返した時は受診して下さい。

If your symptoms persist, get worse, or get better but then come back, come see me again.

275
精密検査
に進む

普通の写真で異常がある時は、CTによる、より精密な検査に進みます。

If we see an abnormal shadow on the x-ray, we will proceed to a more detailed exam using CT.

276
原因不明熱.
体温計測.
次の受診時

できれば、朝昼晩3回、自分の体温を定期的に測って、次の受診の際に見せて下さい。

If you can, check your temperature three times a day (morning, noon, and evening) regularly and show me the results at your next visit.

277
血圧管理

血圧が高めです。今後、血圧が高くならない(類：上がらない)よう、しっかり管理する必要があります。

Your blood pressure is rather high. Beginning now, we need to make sure that your blood pressure doesn't go up.

278
適正な摂
取水分量

水分を摂り過ぎないことが大切です。一日の尿量は1.5リットル位を目安にしましょう。これ位を保つ(類：維持する)ことができれば水分量は十分です。

You should not drink too much water or fluids. This is important. We need to keep your urine output to less than 1.5 L per day. If you can keep to this, your water intake is fine.

グループNo		
279 インフルエンザ予防. 咳エチケット. 外から帰宅	だれでも、咳をする人はマスクをし、咳をする時には口にハンカチを当てて下さい。外から帰ったら、手洗いとうがいをして下さい。水道の水で十分です。 Everyone who has a cough should wear a mask, and cover their mouth with a handkerchief. Be sure to wash your hands and gargle when you come indoors. Tap water is ok.	
280 片頭痛. 除外診断. 経過観察	片頭痛の発作は、繰り返し起きます。しかし他の病気の可能性を除外する必要があります。今後、この点に留意しながら経過をみます。 Migraine attacks can come and go, but we need to rule out other possibilities, by following up in your treatment.	
281 検脈. 持続時間.	次に動悸を感じたら、1分当たりの脈の数を数え、乱れていないかどうかをみ、持続時間を測って下さい。 When you have palpitations next time, please count your pulse per minute. Please also check if your pulse is regular and record the duration of the palpitation.	
282 単純Ｘ線写真. 撮影方向	レントゲン写真は後ろからと、横からと、斜めから、合計3枚撮ります。 I will take x-rays from your back, side, and diagonally, for a total of 3.	
283 疾患特異物質	心筋梗塞で血液中に増える物質があります。これが増えているか検査をしたいと思います。 There is a substance that increases in the blood with myocardial infarction or heart attack. I would like to check the level of this substance.	
284 結核菌塗抹検査. 感染予防措置	仮に結核でも、痰の塗抹検査で結核菌が見つからなければ、他人にうつす可能性は小さいです。もし結核菌が見つかれば、感染防止措置をとる必要が出てきます。 Even if you have tuberculosis, it's unlikely that you will transmit the disease to other people unless the TB organism is found in a sputum smear examination. If the TB organisms are found, we will need to practice infection prevention.	
285 気管支鏡下生検	いくつかの検査をしても診断がつかない時は、直接、気管支鏡で、細胞や組織を採る必要があります。 If it remains undiagnosed after some exams, we need to pick cells or tissue directly using a bronchoscope.	

Phrase

286
グループNo
治療に専念.
去痰剤.
気長に構える

治療に専念しましょう. 痰を軟らかくし, 出しやすくする薬を処方します. 気長に構えましょう.

Let's focus on treatment. I will prescribe some medicine to thin the sputum and make it easier to bring up. With time, you'll get better.

287
ソ経ヘルニア.
大変な手術.
外来・入院
費用.
保証

病名は鼠径ヘルニアです. それほど大変な手術ではありません. しかしもちろん, 手術が100%安全だという保証はありません. 外来費用と入院費用を合わせて12万円位はかかります.

You have an inguinal hernia. The surgery is not difficult, but of course, nothing is 100% guaranteed. The total cost for both outpatient and inpatient care is about 120,000 yen.

288
吐き通し.
点滴する.
模様を見る.
鎮吐剤

今朝から吐き通しとのことですので, 点滴をしましょうか. しかし, 少しずつでも, 十分な量を飲めるなら, そうして模様をみるのも一法です. 二日分の吐き気止めを処方します.

You said you've been throwing up since this morning. Perhaps some i.v. fluids would help, but another choice would be to simply drink enough fluid, even little by little, and see if that helps. I'll prescribe two days worth of anti-nausea medicine.

289
スポーツ
飲料.
スープの
上澄み

スポーツ飲料やスープの上澄みなどを飲んで下さい. 水分は一度にたくさん飲まないで, 少しずつ, 数回に分けて飲んで下さい.

You should drink sports drinks or clear soup, but don't drink too fast or too much at one time. Drink a little bit several times per day.

290
胆石破砕.
衝撃波.
腹腔鏡下
手術

胆石が悪さをしています. 侵襲の大きい手術を考える前に, まず, 衝撃波で石を砕いたり腹腔鏡で取り出すことができるか, やってみましょう.

Your problem is due to a gallstone. Let's try first to break up the stone with ultrasonic waves or to take it out laparoscopically, before considering more invasive surgery.

291
胆のう炎治
療食指示

脂っこい物を食べると痛みが強くなるので, 控えて下さい.

Please avoid fatty foods, as they make your pain worse.

292
自尿観察.
尿路結石

尿と一緒に石が出て来ないか, 排尿時に注意深く見ていて下さい.

Please pay attention when you urinate. You may actually see a stone come out.

グループ No		
293 予約日取得, 二回分の予約	結果が分かるのは、器械を返却してから一週間後です．今日は、検査(類：検査の予約)と、結果説明(類：結果説明の予約)の、二回分の予約をして下さい．	
	We will know the result 1 week after you return the monitor. Please make 2 appointments today for the next exam and an explanation of the results.	
294 次回予約日	私はあなたの次の予約を来週月曜日にとります．	
	I'll make an appointment for you for next Monday.	
295 診断書用紙, 提出期限, 抗体価, 母子手帳	診断書は、会社が必要とする(類：要求する)項目を満たさなくてはなりません．会社が指定する用紙は持っていますか，当院の用紙を使っていいですか．提出期限はいつですか．麻疹の抗体価を調べるには、最低一週間必要です．いつどんな予防接種を受けたかを知るため、母子健康手帳を借りてきて下さい．	
	The medical certification should fulfill the requirement by the company. Do you have the form specified by the company? May I use our form? When is the due date of submission? We need at least 1 week to examine the antibody level of measles. In order to know when and what kind of immunization shots you had, we need you to borrow your mother-child notebook.	
296 自宅療養 期間, 職場復帰	診断書には、自宅療養期間、つまり職場に復帰できる時期を書けばいいですか．	
	Should I write the duration of recuperation at home, which suggests when you can return to work in this medical certificate?	
297 秘守義務, 保険会社, 同意書, 電話説明	私にはあなたの情報を守秘する義務があります．もし職場の人が問い合わせて来たら、だれにだったら、あなたの病状を説明していいですか．基本的に、電話では説明しません．保険会社の人だと、自分の病気についてその人に説明することを許可するという、患者さんの同意書を持って来ます．	
	We must maintain your information as confidential. To whom in your office may I explain your disease condition if someone from your office asks? Basically, we don't talk about the patients' disease condition by phone. There may be a person from the insurance company who brings a consent form for the patient which allows me to explain his/her disease condition to that person.	

Phrase

Chapter-7 ······ 看護過程 nursing process

グループNo

298
検温

体温を測ります．体温計を腋の下にはさんで下さい．

I'd like to check your temperature. Please place this thermometer in your armpit.

299
事後説明，
採血室，
レントゲン室，
理学療法室

この後，血液検査(レントゲン検査，リハビリ)があります．廊下の黄色い線を辿って行き，採血室(レントゲン室，理学療法室，処置室，待合室)の前でお待ち下さい．看護師(レントゲン技師，理学療法士)がお呼びします．

After this, you'll have a blood exam (x-ray exam, rehabilitation). Please, go to the room for blood sampling (x-ray room, room for physiotherapy, treatment room, waiting room) following the yellow line in the corridor, and wait there. A nurse (x-ray technician, physiotherapist) will call you.

300
移動介助，
ストレッ
チャー，
かけ声

ストレッチャーからベッドに移りますね．私たちがシーツごと持ち上げます．いいですか．移りますよ．イチ，ニノ，サン．

We have to move you from the stretcher to the bed. We'll lift you together with the sheet. Are you ready? Here we go -- one, two, three. Oomph.

301
移動介助，
車椅子，
かけ声

車椅子からベッドに移っていただきます．先ず，私の肩に手を回して，つかまって下さい．私は腰を持ちます．ヨーイショ．お尻をベッドに載せて下さい．次に，私が膝を下から抱え，お尻を中心にして，身体を回します．靴を脱ぎますね．仰向けになって下さい．頭を上げて下さい．枕を入れます．はい，下ろして下さい．

Let us help you move from the wheel chair to the bed. First, hold on to me with your arms around my shoulders. I'll grasp your lower back. Good. Place your hip on the bed. Next, I'll turn you, lifting your knees from underneath with your hip as a pivot. Let me take your shoes off. Lie down. Raise your head a bit, so I can put a pillow under your head. Now lower your head. Good.

41

グループNo		
302 体格.腹囲	身長、体重、腹囲を教えて下さい．腹囲は臍の高さに巻き尺(類：メジャー)を当てて測ります．	

Could you tell me your height, weight, and waist size? You can measure it by using a tape measure at the height of your bellybutton.

303 静脈採血. 利き手. 乳癌手術歴. 駆血帯	利き手はどっちですか．右利きでしたら左腕を出して下さい．片方の乳がんの手術を受けましたか．それでは反対側の腕を出して下さい．ゴムで腕を縛ります．親指を中にして、手を軽く握って下さい．それでは針を刺します．チクッとします．痛みは指先に響きますか．	

Which is your dominant hand? If right, give me your left arm. Have you ever had surgery for breast cancer on one side? Then give me your other arm. I'll put a rubber band on your arm. Please make a light fist with your thumb inside. Now I'll insert a needle. You'll feel a slight pin prick. Does the pain travel to your fingertips?

304 静脈採血. 血管が細い. 見えにくい. 前回採血 部位	血管が細く見えにくいです．前回はどこから採りました(類：採血しました)か．血管に入りました．5ml採血します．手を開いて下さい．縛ったゴムを外しますからそのままでいて下さい．これで終わりました．	

It looks like your vessels are thin and difficult to find. Where did the nurse draw blood from before? OK. I've got a vessel. I'll take a 5 ml blood sample. Open your fist. Please don't move your arm, I'll release the band. Now we're finished.

305 採血失敗. 看護師交替. 圧迫止血	すみません、失敗しました．別の看護師に代わります．その間この酒精綿で、私が"いいです"と言うまで、押さえていて下さい．	

Excuse me. This didn't work out. I will ask a colleague to come and help draw blood. Meantime, please hold this cotton pad until I say "OK".

Phrase

306
グループNo
同日他科受診．
他科宛紹介状．
午後の診察

内科診察の後、婦人科を受診していただきます．先生が婦人科宛の紹介状を書いておきます．受け付け窓口で、改めて受診の受付をし、診察室の前でお待ち下さい．午後の診察は3時に始まります．その前に、昼食をとって下さい．

After an examination by the internist, we'd like you to see an OB-GYN doctor, to whom your doctor will have made a referral. Please register for an exam at the reception window and wait in front of the consultation room. Afternoon exams begin at 3. Please have lunch before then.

307
吐物処置．
寒気対策．
酸素吸入

吐き気は治まりましたか．吐きたい時はここに吐いて下さい．大丈夫、気にならないで下さい．汚れたシーツは後で片付けますから．寒いですか．毛布をもう一枚かけましょうか．鼻から酸素を吸っていただきます．

Has your nausea gone away? If you need to throw up, it's ok; you can do it here. We'll clean up any mess. Do you feel cold? Would you like another blanket? Please inhale oxygen from your nose.

308
検査日．
大腸カメラ
検査．
予約が一杯

大腸カメラの検査日は木曜日の午後です．いつがいい(類：都合がいい)ですか．あいにく、その日はもう予約が一杯です．

Colonoscopies are done on Thursday afternoons here. When would be convenient for you? Unfortunately, that date is booked.

309
前処置．
前日の夜．
当日の朝．
検査所要時間

大腸カメラの前に腸を空にする必要があります．前日(類：前の日)の夜は線維の多い物を食べないで下さい．当日の朝、粉末の下剤を2リットルの水に溶かし、1度に200mlずつ、数時間かけて飲みます．水のような便が何回か出て、最後は下剤だけの便になります．検査はおよそ10分で終わり(類：済み)ます．

Before the colonoscopy, you need to empty your bowel. The night before, you should not eat fibrous food, and the morning of the exam you should dissolve this powdered laxative in 2 L of water, and drink one glass (200 ml) at a time over several hours. You will have watery diarrhea several times, but eventually just water will come out. The exam itself is about 10 min.

310 浣腸, 口呼吸, 排便我慢	浣腸します．お尻の力を抜き、口でゆっくり、息をして下さい．液を入れて数分経つと (類：後に) トイレに行きたくなります．浣腸液が役に立つように，できるだけ我慢してから排便して下さい． Let me give you an enema. Relax your bottom, and breathe slowly through your mouth. After a couple of minutes, you'll feel the need for having a bowel movement. Please wait as long as possible before having a bowel movement, so that the enema fluid will help.
311 診療の順番, 苦情対応	私の順番はまだですか．もう一時間待っています．あなたの順番は次の次です．私よりおそく来た人が，先に呼ばれている．お待たせして申し訳ございません． *Is my turn yet? I have been waiting for 1 hour.* Your turn is the one after next. *That person came later than me, but was called before me.* We apologize to have kept you waiting.
312 診察終了, 異常時指示	これで今日の診察が終わりました．このファイルを、会計窓口に出して (類：持って行って) 下さい．お大事にして下さい．具合が思わしくない時は，次の予約日まで待たないで，いつでもおいで下さい (類：受診して下さい)．病院は 24 時間受け付けますので． I think we're finished here today. Please take this folder to the receptionist. Take care of yourself. If you don't feel well, don't wait for your next appointment. Come and see me any time. The hospital is open 24 hrs.
313 予約制, 予約無し患者, 当日受診	予約無し (類：予約無しの患者) でも受け付けますが、通常の診療は原則的に予約制です．当日受診の場合でも、前もって電話で予約して下さい．そうしないと，待たなくてはなりません． We can accept walk-ins, but regular office visits are usually by appointment. Even if it's for a same day visit, please call ahead. Otherwise you will have to wait.

Phrase

Chapter-8 …… その他 others

グループ No

314
診療科医呼称

眼科の、胸部外科の、形成外科の、外科の、呼吸器科の、耳鼻科の、循環器科の、消化器科の、小児科の、心臓外科の、心療内科の、精神科の、内科の、内分泌科の、脳外科の、泌尿器科の、皮膚科の、腹部外科の、婦人科の、放射線科の、麻酔科の医者

ophthalmologist, thoracic surgeon, plastic surgeon, surgeon, pulmonologist (or: lung doctor), ENT doctor, cardiologist, gastroenterologist (or: gastrointestinal doctor), pediatrician, cardiac surgeon, psychologist, psychiatrist, internist, endocrinologist, brain surgeon, urologist, dermatologist, abdominal surgeon, gynecologist (or: OB/GYN doctor), radiologist, anesthesiologist

315
診察の順番

受け付けで一列に並んで下さい。番号順に呼びます。

Please form a line at the reception window (or: desk). We will call you in numeric order.

316
健康保険証、自費診療、返金、自己負担分

健康保険証は、その月の最初の受診の時に、必ず持って来て下さい。持って来ない場合は、受診が自費になるので、注意して下さい。後で持って来れば返金(払い戻し)します。あなたの自己負担分は3割です。

Please make sure you bring your health insurance card on the first visit of the month. Please note that the visit will be at your own expense if you don't bring that. We will refund the money if you bring it later. Your self-pay ratio is 30 percent.

317
調剤薬局、薬代、調剤料

処方箋を渡します。近くの調剤薬局で調剤してもらって下さい。薬局では、薬代と調剤料が請求されます。

We will give you a prescription. Please fill it at your nearest dispensing pharmacy. You will be charged a drug and preparation fee at the pharmacy.

INDEX

グループNo 数字

287	100% 安全だという保証はない	nothing is 100% guaranteed
74	24 時間風呂	Does your home bath have a 24 hour system
248	24 時間記録する	record your ECG over 24 hours
312	24 時間受け付ける	The hospital is open 24 hrs.

英語

258	CT 検査をする	do a contrast CT
249	CT 写真は (この)	This CT picture shows
275	CT による検査	exam using CT
242	MR 画像では	In an MR image
242	MR 血管画像では	In this MR angiogram image

あ

171	アーッと声を出す	say "Ahhh"
213	間 (説明の)	during the explanation
133	間は (電柱と電柱の)	the distance between electrical poles
308	あいにくその日は	Unfortunately, that date is
7	仰向けに倒れる	fell down on his back
202	仰向けに寝る	lie down on your back
204	仰向けに戻る	Turn back over and lie on your back.
301	仰向けになる	Lie down.
131	赤い色のついた食べ物	red or brown colored food
22	赤く腫れている (おでこが)	is red and feels hot and swollen
52	上がらない (脚が)	can't lift my right leg
230	上がり方 (血糖値の)	the response to an oral glucose drink
277	上がる (血圧が)	go up
198	アキレス腱反射	your Achilles tendon reflex
262	悪性の嚢胞性陰影	The malignant cystic shadow
237	上げ下げする (脚を)	move your legs up and down
206	上げる (脚を)	lift your leg
180	上げる (腕を)	Raise your right arm
173	あごを引く	tuck in your chin
62	あざができる	got a purplish bruise
211	朝は (受診当日の)	beginning the morning of your visit
276	朝昼晩 3 回	three times a day (morning, noon, and evening)
19	味 (物の)	its taste

47

52	脚が上がらない	can't lift my right leg
51	脚が痛くなる	My legs hurt
75	味がいつもと違う	sensed an unusual taste
202	足首まで	to the ankle
57	足腰に力が入らない	My legs feel weak.
237	足腰の筋力の衰え	muscle weakness in your legs and lower body
98	味付けは	seasoning in food
38	脚の付け根に	in my armpit (groin, neck)
46	脚の付け根が膨らんでいる	have a bulge in my groin
197	脚を下げる	let your legs hang down
85	汗かきだ	sweat a lot
69	暖かさ	warmth
112	頭の片側だけ(痛むのは)	Does it hurt just on one side of your head?
115	頭のどこが痛みますか	Where in your head does it hurt?
241	頭の中に	in your brain
301	頭を上げる	Raise your head
148	辺りが(みぞおち)	around the pit of your stomach
213	辺りに(喉仏の)	around your Adam's apple
281	当たりの脈の数(一分)	your pulse per minute
23	当たる(ボールが頭に)	A ball hit me on the head.
240	圧痛がある(甲状腺に)	You have thyroid tenderness
116	合っている(眼鏡が)	Is the correction proper?
137	圧迫感(胸の)	pressure in your chest
302	当てて(巻尺を~に)	by using a tape measure at ~
306	宛の紹介状(婦人科)	to whom your doctor will have made a referral
129	当てはまるか言う(どれに)	Describe the phlegm you see.
205	当てる(音叉を踝に)	place a tuning fork on your ankle
279	当てる(口にハンカチを)	cover their mouth with a handkerchief
209	痕ですか(何の手術の)	What kind of surgery was that for?
161	後でも(排尿をした)	even after you finish
316	後で持って来れば	if you bring it later
220	後で読んで下さい	read them carefully later
70	あなたの言うめまい	your dizziness

48

INDEX

137	あなたの言う動悸は~	When you say "palpitation", do you mean ~
129	あなたの痰	the phlegm you see
98	脂っこい物	oily or fatty food
291	脂っこい物	fatty foods
12	甘い物	sweet things
178	あまり心配いらない	Things are probably o.k.
256	あまり心配しないで	don't worry too much
267	洗い流す	wash out
212	あり得る(ということも)	it is possible that
243	ある(~する薬が)	We have two medicines
260	ある(熱が出る他の病気に~が)	One of the other diseases with fever and right-side lower stomach pain is ~
283	ある(~で~に増える物質が)	There is a substance that increases in ~ with ~
232	ある(疑いが)	There is a possibility that
250	ある(影が)	There is a markedly white shadow
232	ある(簡単な検査が)	there is a simple, easy exam
237	ある(簡単な運動が)	There are some simple exercises
209	ある(傷痕が)	I see you have a 5 cm scar
96	ある(休肝日が)	Are there days when you don't drink any?
247	ある(~という所見が)	There is a finding called ~
299	ある(レントゲン検査が)	you'll have a blood exam (x-ray exam
50	歩くとよろめく	when walking
64	ある程度の物忘れ	Some level of forgetfulness
129	アレルギー性の	may be due to an allergy
287	合わせて~円だ	The total cost for ~ is ~ yen.
60	合わない(化粧品が)	had an allergic reaction to this cosmetic
138	安静時に	resting
233	安静だけで	simply resting is enough to get well
132	安静にすると	after you rest
225	安定剤	some antidepressants

い

273	いい(~して)	you can return to school
271	いい(~するのが)	You should go see
224	いい(~薬が)	I recommend some medicine for ~
213	いい(同席するのが)	It would be helpful if

49

224	いい (寝つきが)	you may fall asleep quickly
144	いい (腹の具合は)	Does your stomach now feel all right?
297	いいですか (説明して)	may I explain
300	いいですか	Are you ready?
308	いいですか (都合が)	When would be convenient for you?
305	いいですと言うまで (私が)	until I say "OK"
219	いい (塗抹検査と)	is called smear examination
129	言う (どれに当てはまるか)	Describe the phlegm
141	いう薬 (ニトロールと)	the medicine called "Nitorol"
247	いう所見 (〜と)	a finding called " Dissection"
109	いうより〜 (痛いと)	〜 rather than simply hurting
80	言えば (食あたりと)	Speaking of food poisoning
215	以外のことは (〜)	activities except that you cannot 〜
208	以外のどこかに (口)	elsewhere other than your mouth
84	以外の病気 (〜)	any illness lasting more than a week other than 〜
269	以下の赤血球 (4個)	there were less than 4 red blood cells
162	勢いは (尿の)	your urine flow rate
135	息が切れる	Are you out of breath
110	息が止まる	stop breathing
132	息切れする	When are you short of breath?
132	息切れするのは〜の時だけ	is it only during 〜
256	息切れを感じる	which can make you short of breath
120	息が苦しくなりますか (鼻づまりで)	Any nasal obstruction to breathing?
134	息苦しさ	shortness of breath
136	息苦しく感じる	feel out of breath
179	息をする	breathe
310	息をする (口で)	breathe slowly through your mouth
181	息を吐く (速く)	blow out as fast as possible
74	行く (公衆浴場に)	Have you been to a public bath
228	行く (耳鼻科に)	see an ENT (ear, nose, throat) doctor
310	行く (トイレに)	having a bowel movement
6	意識がはっきりしない	My father seems alert but a bit confused.
278	維持する (これ位を)	keep your urine output to
216	異常陰影	abnormal shadows
275	異常がある (普通の写真で)	see an abnormal shadow on the x-ray

50

INDEX

68	異常な感じ	unusual feeling
245	異常な呼吸音	a possibly abnormal sound
272	以上の熱がある時(摂氏38度)	When you have temperature greater than 38 degrees Centigrade
145	胃食道逆流	gastroesophageal reflux disease
48	以前、椎間板ヘルニアに	I had a slipped disc before
139	以前にも	before
48	痛い(腰が)	My lower back hurts
18	痛い(喉の奥が)	My throat's sore way in the back.
106	痛い(飲み込む時に)	Does it hurt to swallow?
160	痛い(排尿時に)	Does it hurt when you urinate?
113	痛い(耳が)	Do you have any pain in your ears?
148	痛い(みぞおち辺りが)	Did it hurt around the pit of your stomach
183	痛い時は	when it hurts
43	痛い所が	the joint soreness
106	痛いところはありますか(〜で)	Do you have any soreness inside 〜
192	痛かったら(押されて)	if it hurts when I press down
46	痛くなる(時に)	Sometimes it hurts.
301	いただきます(〜して)	Let us help you move
141	痛みは治まる	Does the pain stop
291	痛みが強くなる	make your pain worse
265	痛み止め	a painkiller
106	痛みますか(喉のどの辺りが)	Where in your throat is it sore?
140	痛みますか(胸のどこが)	Where does it hurt in your chest?
160	痛みを感じる(〜する時に)	feel pain when 〜
108	痛むのは〜ですか	Is it in the back of your throat
111	傷める(首を)	had a neck injury
140	痛んでいる(今も)	Is it painful now?
238	一因だ(タバコも)	Smoking may contribute to this
240	一時的に	temporarily
269	一視野に(顕微鏡の)	in one microscopic field
309	一度に200 mlずつ	one glass (200 ml) at a time
289	一度にたくさん	too much at one time
197	イチ・ニ・サン・ハイと	"One, two, three, go"
265	一日3回飲む薬	to be taken regularly three times per day

51

130	一日に	in a day
300	イチ、ニノ、サン	one, two, three. Oomph.
216	一枚の写真に	In one conventional image
73	いつ起きましたか (～は)	When did the dizziness start?
308	いつがいいですか	When would be convenient for you?
131	一緒に (咳と)	when you coughed
112	一旦起きると	once it starts
183	言って下さい (痛い時は)	please let me know when it hurts
195	言って下さい (痛かったら)	tell me if it hurts
153	いつですか (最後の生理は)	When was your last period?
165	いつですか (～を指摘されたのは)	When was it first pointed out to you that ～
295	いつですか (期限は)	When is the due date
312	いつでもおいで下さい	Come and see me any time.
295	いつどんな予防接種を	when and what kind of immunization shots
308	一杯だ (その日は予約が)	that date is booked
288	一法だ (～するのも)	another choice would be to simply drink
215	いつも通りの生活	your daily routine
215	いつも通りする	perform all your normal daily activities
75	いつもと違う (味が)	sensed an unusual taste
211	いつも飲んでいる薬	your usual medicines
148	移動する (痛みが)	did the pain move to
237	いながら (椅子にかけて)	while sitting
261	胃にポリープ	a polyp in the stomach
101	居眠り運転が原因だ	because of being drowsy
101	居眠りする	doze off
149	胃の検査	stomach checkup
149	胃の検査をカメラでする	have a barium contrast x-ray, or a gastric camera exam for stomach checkup
110	いびきをかく	you snore
166	イボのような物	a hemorrhoid
176	今から～する	Now I'm going to examine
190	今から～する	Now I'll check
195	今から叩く	I'm going to tap you
144	今は腹の具合はいい	Does your stomach now feel all right?
253	意味する (～を)	This means ～
94	いる (同じ症状の人が)	Are there any family members

52

INDEX

254	いる (結核菌が)	there is a tuberculosis organism
266	入れる (栄養分を)	give you nutrition
196	入れる (お尻に指を)	insert my finger into your anus
301	入れる (枕を)	put a pillow under your head
216	色々なものが重なって	many different organs, all overlapped
131	色のついた (赤や茶の)	red or brown colored food
42	違和感がある	have a funny feeling
161	いわゆる残尿感	a sensation called "constant urge to urinate"
143	言われた (検査を受けるように)	you were told to have
93	言われたことはないですか (〜と)	Have you ever had 〜
102	言われたことはありますか (〜と)	Have you ever been told that 〜
117	言われる (むくんだと)	Has anyone told you
254	陰影から	from the shadow
252	陰影の濃さ	This shadow
208	陰部に (たとえば)	such as your pubic area
236	インフルエンザ	Flu

う

236	うがいが大切	gargling
279	うがいをする	gargle
315	受け付けで	at the reception window (or: desk)
312	受け付ける	The hospital is open
313	受け付ける (予約無しでも)	accept walk-ins
306	受け付けをする (受診の)	register for an exam
303	受けましたか (〜の手術を)	Have you ever had surgery for 〜
83	受ける (インフルエンザの予防接種を)	had a flu shot
220	受ける (気管支鏡検査を)	have a bronchoscopic exam
165	受ける (精密検査を)	have a thorough examination
47	受ける (二次検診を)	get a second medical check
138	動かす時 (身体を)	when you are exercising
237	動きを少なくする	be inactive
108	後ろ (首の)	in the back of the neck

53

201	後ろ足のつま先を前足の踵につけて	with the toes of the back foot touching the heel of the front one
206	後ろが痛む(腿の)	does the back of your thigh hurt
190	後ろから	from behind
282	後ろから撮る	take x-rays from your back
190	後に立って検査する	check some signs, standing behind you
107	後ろを伝って(涎が喉の)	down the back of my throat
185	後ろを向く	turn around
232	疑いがある(〜の)	There is a possibility that you have sleep apnea.
249	疑いが濃い	we strongly suspect
258	疑いがある(〜の)	There is a possibility that you have appendicitis.
238	疑われる(〜や〜が)	This is likely either 〜 or 〜
234	打ち勝つ力	your strength
208	内側に(唇の)	inside your lip
284	うつす(他人に病気を)	transmit the disease to other people
301	移っていただきます(ベッドに)	Let us help you move
300	移りますよ	Here we go --
43	移る(痛い所が)	the joint soreness moves around
300	移りますね(ベッドに)	We have to move you
59	腕にしみのようなものが	age spot or liver spot on my arm
303	腕を出す(反対側の)	give me your other arm
252	ウニのとげ	sea urchin spines
289	上澄み(スープの)	clear soup
37	膿んでいる(おできが)	it has pus in it
237	運動(役に立つ)	exercises that will help
226	うんと気になる	you're really worried

え

253	鋭角だ	an acute (obtuse) angle
242	影響(脳梗塞の)	the effects of a stroke
266	栄養分を入れる	give you nutrition
268	液体が溜まる	accumulation of fluid
247	枝分かれる(心臓から)	it branches out from the heart
239	炎症(扁桃腺の)	The inflammation (infection) in your tonsil
260	炎症(壁の凹みの)	inflammation of a small pit-like structure

INDEX

お

79	置いておく	left them at room temperature
312	おいで下さい	Come and see me
173	追う(指先を眼で)	Follow my finger with your eyes
131	嘔吐と一緒に	when you coughed (vomited)
270	多い(〜することが)	most of them have normal urine
154	多い(生理が)	Are your periods heavy?
249	多い(良性疾患に)	is common with benign diseases
110	大いびきで	because of your loud snoring
243	多い病気だ(女性に)	is common among young women
253	大きい(角度が)	is smaller (bigger)
181	大きく息を吸う	Take a deep breath in
262	大きくなる(陰影が)	grows rapidly
176	大きさ(瞳の)	the size of your pupils
213	大きさだ(弁当箱位の)	The machine is the size of a bento-box.
112	大きな音	loud sounds
247	大きな血管	the aorta
142	大きな咳をする	coughing violently
95	大きな病気	a serious disease
81	大勢いる(〜の人は)	Are there lots of colds?
272	多目の水分	lots of fluids
102	大笑いする	you were laughing loudly
71	起き上がる時	when waking up
42	起きた時(朝)	when I wake up in the morning
73	起きてから今まで	since it started
142	起きる(痛みが)	this pain happened
112	起きる(頭痛が)	How long does the pain last once it starts?
255	起きる(寝ている状態から)	going from lying down to sitting up
242	起きる(脳梗塞が)	it developed
222	起きる(問題が)	you will encounter more problems
244	置く(舌の下に)	place it under your tongue
108	奥(喉の)	in the back of your throat
18	奥が痛い(喉の)	My throat's sore way in the back.
218	奥から(胸の)	cough up the sputum from your lung
112	奥は痛む(眼の)	behind your eyes
100	奥まで吸い込む(タバコは)	deeply

55

154	おくれる (生理は)	Is your period irregular or late?
198	起こし (上半身を)	with your upper body upright
264	起こす (胆嚢炎を)	it causes cholecystitis
257	起こすことがあるので(〜を)	because of potential 〜
220	抑える (咳と吐き気を)	prevent coughing and gagging
305	押さえる (酒精綿で)	hold this cotton pad
141	治まる (痛みは)	Does the pain stop
147	治まる (それは)	pain that goes away
307	治まる (吐き気が)	Has your nausea gone away?
192	押されて痛かったら	if it hurts when I press down
91	教えて下さい (薬を)	please tell me which ones
192	教えて下さい (痛かったら)	Tell me if it hurts
196	お尻に指を入れる	insert my finger into your anus
310	お尻の力を抜く	Relax your bottom
301	お尻をベッドに載せる	Place your hip on the bed.
183	押す (胸を)	push on your chest
193	押す時と	when I press down
311	おそく来た (私より)	came later than me
247	恐らく解離が〜の原因と	this is the likely cause of 〜
312	お大事に	Take care of yourself.
74	お宅のお風呂	your home bath
229	穏やかだ (所見が)	shows relatively mild abnormality
264	落ち込む (胆管に)	falls into biliary duct
4	落ち着かない (気持が)	restless
151	落ち着きがない (腹の)	feel uncomfortable in your stomach
225	落ち着く (気持が)	can help
225	落ち着く (脈が)	bring your pulse rate down
54	落ちてくる (ブロックが)	Some bricks from a wall fell on me
107	落ちて痰になる (伝って)	there's mucus running down the back
37	おできができる	have a pimple on my back
22	おでこが赤い	My forehead is red
40	落とす (食べ物を)	drop food from my chopsticks
237	衰え (筋力の)	muscle weakness
162	同じ (若い時と)	the same as when you were young
220	同じ位 (太さは 〜と)	Its diameter is about the same as
250	同じくらい白い (肋骨と)	as white as ribs
8	同じことを聞き返す	asks the same things repeatedly

56

INDEX

64	同じことを言う	repeat themselves
189	同じことをする	do the same thing
76	同じような症状の人が	coworkers who also have these symptoms
94	同じ症状の人	children, with the same symptoms you have
126	同じ強さだ (咳は)	Is your cough the same
77	同じような症状	similar symptoms
113	同じように聞こえる (右左で)	hear equally well in both ears
152	おならが出る	have gas
215	お風呂	take a bath
9	覚えられない	can't recall recent things
311	お待たせして申し訳ない	We apologize to have kept you waiting
299	お待ちください (〜の前で)	wait there
20	重い (頭が)	My head feels heavy.
78	思い当たることがある (〜について)	Do you think there's a chance of 〜
65	重い感じ (痛みは)	dull and heavy
9	思い出す	can remember things of the past
75	思いつかない (悪くなっているとは)	I had no idea that it had gone bad
233	思う (風邪を引いただけだと)	I suspect you just have a common cold.
268	思う (浣腸が効くと)	I suggest an enema will help.
36	重苦しい (背中が)	feel heaviness in my back
147	重苦しい痛み	dull pain
312	思わしくない (具合が)	don't feel well
303	親指を中にして	with your thumb inside
99	およそ何本	About how many cigarettes
239	及ぶ (炎症が周囲に)	affecting the surrounding tissue
112	降りる (階段を)	walking down stairs
301	下ろす (頭を)	lower your head
196	終わった (はい)	Now it's done.
312	終わった (診察が)	I think we're finished
309	終わる (およそ10分で)	The exam itself is about 10 min.
153	終わる (生理が)	My period started (finished)
160	終わる (排尿を)	when you are about to finish
205	音叉を踝に当てる	place a tuning fork on your ankle

か

255	臥位から〜位になる	going from lying down to sitting up
101	会議中に	during conferences or meetings
312	会計窓口に	to the receptionist
215	解釈する	interpret the results
255	改善する(起きると)	improves when
24	階段を踏み外す	tripped on some stairs
136	階段を上がる	climbing up a hill or stairs
306	書いておく(紹介状を)	will have made a referral
293	回分の予約をする(二)	make 2 appointments
261	外来で	in the out-patient clinic
287	外来費用	cost for both outpatient and inpatient care
247	解離という所見	a finding called "Dissection"
68	会話が難しい	have difficulty making conversation
101	会話中に	when you are talking
3	顔色が悪い	looks pale
173	顔を動かす	moving your head
190	顔を左に向ける	Turn your head to the left.
301	抱える(膝を下から)	lifting your knees from underneath
196	抱える(両膝を両手で)	hold your knees with both hands
84	かかったことがある(病気に)	Have you had any illness
87	かかっていた(別の医者に)	Have you seen another doctor
87	かかっていた(別の病院に)	been to another hospital
199	踵で立つ	Stand on your heels
55	踵の高い靴	high heels
200	踵とつま先をくっつけて(左右の)	with heels and toes touching each other
271	かかりつけの皮膚科	your dermatologist
219	かかる(8週間)	it will take 8 weeks
95	かかる(大きな病気に)	Have you ever had a serious disease
213	かかる(説明に20〜30分)	the explanation will be 20-30 minutes
132	かかる(何時間も)	Does it take
220	書かれている(〜は説明書に)	〜 are in the booklet
79	かきを生で食べる	eat raw oysters
228	書く(紹介状を)	give you a referral
296	書く(診断書に)	write

58

INDEX

253	角度 (胸膜と陰影のなす)	The angle between ~ and ~
309	かけて (数時間)	over several hours
101	欠ける (集中力が)	have trouble concentrating
182	かける (タオルを)	cover yourself with this towel
307	かける (毛布を)	Would you like another blanket?
216	重なって見える (色々なものが)	see many different organs, all overlapped
232	貸し出す (器機を)	I will lend you a machine
190	貸して下さい (手を)	give me your hand
240	過剰になっている (~が)	have excessive thyroid hormone
152	ガスが出る	have gas
27	霞がかかっている (眼に)	My vision is blurry.
266	ガスを抜く (管で)	relieve your gas with a tube
124	風邪で学校を休む	absent in elementary school due to colds
234	風邪などのウィルス	viruses such as the common cold
81	風邪を引いている人は大勢	lots of colds
86	風邪を引いたら	When you have a cold
281	数える (脈の数を)	count your pulse
77	家族のなかに~がいる	Does your family have ~
201	片足で立つ	stand on one foot
127	硬い (痰は)	thick
39	肩が凝る	My shoulder feels stiff (or: I have a stiff shoulder)
17	片側から (口の)	from one side of my mouth
112	片側だけ (痛むのは頭の)	Does it hurt just on one side of your head?
122	硬さ (洟の)	the consistency of any nasal discharge
307	片付ける	We'll clean up any mess.
301	肩に手を回して (私の)	with your arms around my shoulders
201	片方の足をもう片方の足の後に置いて立つ	stand with one foot behind the other
202	片方の脚を上げる	Lift up one leg
150	がち (腹は緩み)	tend to have soft stools
82	学級閉鎖をする	just some classes
82	学校全体が休校する	Was the whole school closed
273	学校に行く	return to school

59

270	活動すると	after exercise
153	月 16 日に (11)	on November 16
254	かどうか見る (〜)	see whether there is
281	かどうかをみる(乱れていない)	check if your pulse is regular
241	過度の緊張	excessive muscle strain
102	金縛りになる	being paralyzed
271	必ず〜して下さい	Make sure you go see
316	必ず〜して下さい	Please make sure you 〜
46	かなり前	a while ago
129	可能性が高い(炎症の)	may be due to
153	可能性はある(妊娠の)	Do you think you might be pregnant?
239	可能性がある(〜の)	an abscess is possible
280	可能性(他の病気の)	other possibilities
284	可能性が小さい(うつす)	it's unlikely that
156	下腹部が痛む	Does your lower abdomen hurt
61	かぶれる(絆創膏に)	had a funny skin reaction to the Band-Aid
95	花粉症はどうですか	How about hay fever
267	我慢する(排尿を)	hold back or wait too long to urinate
310	我慢する(できるだけ)	wait as long as possible
244	噛む	chew
149	カメラでする(胃の検査を)	have a barium contrast x-ray, or a gastric camera exam for stomach checkup
168	痒い(それは)	Is your rash itchy?
31	痒くなる(眼が)	my eyes and nose are itchy
224	痒み止め	anti-itch medicine
271	痒み止め	some anti-itch medicine
224	痒みのために	due to cough or itchiness
126	空咳だ(咳は)	Is your cough dry
213	身体に付けるセンサー	sensors attached to your body
248	身体に付ける(記録器を)	wear a small monitor
138	身体を動かす	exercising
236	身体を休める	getting enough rest
309	空にする(腸を)	empty your bowel
229	カリウムが少ない	potassium is low
295	借りてくる	borrow
73	軽い(症状がより)	is it better now

60

INDEX

256	軽くする (症状を)	lighten your symptoms
195	軽く叩く	tap you lightly
240	軽くなる (痛みが)	get better
255	軽くなる (症状が)	your shortness of breath improves
303	軽く握る (手を)	make a light fist
207	軽く曲げる (脚を)	Bend your legs slightly
19	乾いている (眼も)	My eyes are dry
19	乾く (口が)	My mouth is dry
140	変わる (痛みの強さは)	Does the intensity of the pain change?
305	代わる (別の看護師に)	ask a colleague to come and help draw blood
161	感がある (残尿)	feel a sensation called "constant urge to urinate"
290	考える (手術を)	considering more invasive surgery
141	間隔 (痛みの)	the interval between pain episodes
41	感覚がにぶい (手の)	There's a dull or numb sensation in my hand.
314	眼科の医者	ophthalmologist
210	肝機能	liver function
68	感じ (異常な)	unusual feeling
70	感じだ (~しているような)	like riding in a boat
109	感じだ (ヒリヒリする)	Does your throat feel like it's burning
264	関しては (石に)	Regarding the stone
71	感じる (めまいを)	feel dizzy
117	感じる (むくんでいると)	think your face looks puffy
205	感じる (振えを)	sense the vibration
281	感じる (動悸を)	have palpitations
237	感じると (息切れを)	If you're often short of breath
239	感染 (扁桃腺の)	The inflammation (infection) in your tonsil
231	感染症か腫瘍か	if this is an infection or a tumor
284	感染防止措置	infection prevention
232	簡単な検査	a simple, easy exam
268	浣腸が効くと思う	an enema will help
310	浣腸する	give you an enema
310	浣腸液	enema fluid
277	管理する必要がある	we need to make sure that

き

114	キーッという高い音	a high pitched squealing sound
121	黄色っぽい (痰の色は)	Yellowish
144	黄色っぽい	yellowish
135	着替え	such as changing clothes
80	気がする (生焼きだった)	I remember
296	期間 (自宅療養の)	the duration of recuperation at home
285	気管支鏡で	using a bronchoscope
249	気管支 (黒い影は)	a bronchial tube or airway
8	聞き返す (同じことを)	asks the same things repeatedly
303	利き手はどっちですか	Which is your dominant hand?
323	効く (安定剤を飲むと)	some antidepressants can help
81	聞く (休校したと)	I recently heard that
83	効く (健康保険が)	Health insurance doesn't cover immunization shots.
265	効く (整腸剤が)	will help
178	聴く (胸の音を)	listen to your breathing
295	期限 (提出の)	the due date of submission
257	危険だ (〜ので)	dangerous because of ~
113	聞こえる (右左で同じように)	you hear
245	聞こえる (異常な呼吸音が)	I hear
246	聞こえる (雑音が)	I hear
255	起座位になる (〜位から)	going from lying down to sitting up
212	技師の条件設定	the machine settings
209	傷痕 (5 センチの)	5 cm scar
265	規則的に飲む薬	to be taken regularly
68	気づく (異常な感じに)	notice this unusual feeling
159	気づく (頻尿に)	notice that you have frequent urination
48	ぎっくり腰のようだ	like I strained it
286	気長に構えましょう	With time, you'll get better.
307	気にしないで下さい	it's ok
226	気になるなら	If you're really worried
1	気分がぱっとしない	don't feel well
234	基本だ (治療の)	Treatment is basically
297	基本的に	Basically
297	義務がある (守秘する)	must maintain
220	決めて下さい (検査を受けるか)	you can decide whether

62

INDEX

12	気持が悪くなる	feel bad
96	休肝日	days when you don't drink any
81	休校する	a school was closed
262	急に大きくなる	grows rapidly
72	急に立ち上がる	suddenly stand up
236	休養すること	getting enough rest
252	境界が明瞭	its edges are sharply defined
133	競争する (だれかと)	if you are not competing with someone
312	今日の診察が終わった	I think we're finished here today.
212	今日の写真に	in today's x-ray
314	胸部外科の医者	thoracic surgeon
247	胸部の検査	the chest examination
253	胸膜に向かって	from the lung towards the pleura
239	強力な抗生剤が必要だ	you'll definitely need an antibiotic
297	許可する (〜について〜に説明することを)	allows me to explain 〜 to 〜
147	キリキリと痛む (それは)	Is it a sharp pain
178	きれい (音は)	Your breath sounds are clear
248	記録器 (心電図)	a small monitor
139	気を失う	blacked out
252	均一な (陰影の濃さが)	This shadow looks pretty uniform
259	緊急の手術が必要だ	You are in urgent need of an operation.
188	ギンギンギラギラするように	twirl your hands around like this
241	筋収縮性頭痛	tension headache
241	緊張 (筋肉の)	muscle strain
237	筋力の衰え (足腰の)	muscle weakness in your legs and lower body

く

312	具合が思わしくない	don't feel well
252	空洞も見える (中に)	can also see the cavity inside
211	空腹時血液検査	take a fasting blood sample
230	空腹時の血糖	a fasting blood sugar exam
230	空腹でなくとも	even without fasting
211	くしゃみが出る	I get the sneezes
119	くしゃみが出る	Do you sneeze often?
317	薬代	a drug and preparation fee
90	薬の説明書	the explanation forms

63

89	薬を処方する	prescribe
11	薬を飲む (〜の)	taking drugs (or: medication) for 〜
290	砕く (石を)	break up the stone
266	管でガスを抜く	relieve your gas with a tube
230	口から飲んだブドウ糖	an oral glucose drink
310	口で息をする	breathe slowly through your mouth
17	口の片側	one side of my mouth
106	口の中で	inside your mouth
170	口元を横に引く	pull your lips sideways
171	口を開ける	Open your mouth
180	くっつく (腕が耳に)	it touches your ear
200	くっつけて (左右の踵とつま先を)	with heels and toes touching each other
301	靴を脱ぎますね	Let me take your shoes off.
38	首にしこりが触れる	in my armpit (groin, neck)
172	首の硬さを診る	examine your neck for stiffness
241	首の周囲の筋肉の緊張	muscle strain around your neck
184	首を前に曲げる	tuck your chin to your chest
260	凹み (大腸の壁の)	a small pit-like structure in the colon
197	組む (両手を)	Hold both hands
278	位を目安にする (〜は 1.5L)	keep 〜 to less than 1.5 L
70	暗くなる (眼の前が)	fainting
222	比べて (〜に)	compared with normal
259	比べて (〜と)	as compared with 〜
280	繰り返し起きる (発作は)	attacks can come and go
207	ぐるっと回って腹這いになる	Turn back over on your stomach
205	踝に当てる (音叉を)	place a tuning fork on your ankle
301	車椅子から	from the wheel chair
215	くれぐれも〜して下さい	Please make sure that 〜
144	黒っぽい	blackish
220	詳しいことは	Detailed explanations
165	詳しく教える (検査について)	tell me the details of the test

け

280	経過をみる	following up in your treatment
139	経験がある (〜の)	Have you ever had 〜
260	憩室炎	colon diverticulitis
314	形成外科の医者	plastic surgeon

INDEX

7	痙攣する	were cramping
314	外科の医者	surgeon
54	怪我をする(脚に)	my leg got hurt
309	下剤を溶かす	dissolve this powdered laxative
60	化粧品	this cosmetic
277	血圧が	Your blood pressure
211	血液検査をする	take a fasting blood sample
258	血液検査をする	do a blood test
299	血液検査がある	you'll have a blood exam
213	血液中の	oxygen level in the blood
283	血液中に増える(心筋梗塞で)	increases in the blood
210	血液で~を調べる	examine the blood for tumor markers
123	血縁者	your blood relatives
229	結果~(検査の)	Your blood chemistry suggests that ~
219	結果が分かる	We will know the result
293	結果が分かるのは一週後だ	We will know the result 1 week after
254	結核菌	a tuberculosis organism
284	結核でも(仮に)	Even if you have tuberculosis
254	結核を否定する	rule out tuberculosis
293	結果説明	an explanation of the results
165	結果はどうしたか	What was the result of the exam?
276	結果を見せて下さい	show me the results
252	血管が	the vessels
257	血管に詰まる	blocking the vessels
304	血管に入る	OK. I've got a vessel.
215	結構だ(いつも通りして)	You can perform
178	結構です(はい)	Good.
241	結構有効だ	may be helpful for
131	血痰が出る	had bloody sputum
165	血尿	bloody urine
145	げっぷがある	you burp or belch
272	解熱剤	a fever reducing medicine
273	解熱する	the fever goes away
152	下痢しがち	tend to have diarrhea
265	下痢止めを	anti-diarrheal medicines
102	蹴るような動きをする	you jerk or kick
224	けれども(~だ)	even though ~

65

101	原因だ(居眠り運転が)	Was it because of being drowsy
247	原因と(解離が〜の)	this is the likely cause of ~
238	原因の一つだ(タバコも)	Smoking may contribute to this
268	原因は(腹痛の)	a cause of your stomach pain
102	幻覚を感じる	had hallucinations
5	元気が出ない	have no energy
316	健康保険証	your health insurance card
149	検査(胃の)	stomach checkup
213	検査技師	A laboratory technician
247	検査をした(造影剤を使って)	We have completed the chest examination
283	検査をしたいと思う(〜か)	I would like to check the level of ~
190	検査する(徴候を)	I'll check some signs
269	検査では	According to today's microscopic examination
229	検査の結果〜	Your blood chemistry suggests that ~
293	検査の予約	appointments today for the next exam
308	検査日は〜曜日の午後だ(大腸カメラの)	Colonoscopies are done on Thursday afternoons
254	検査をする	Let me examine your sputum to see
227	現時点では	At this point
143	健診で	in your medical checkup
47	健診を受ける	had an annual health checkup
143	健診を受ける	have a checkup
269	顕微鏡検査	microscopic examination
222	減量する(5キロ)	You should lose roughly 5 kg.
こ		
98	濃い(味付けは)	like strong seasoning in food
249	濃い(疑いが)	we strongly suspect
282	合計3枚撮る	for a total of 3
124	高校時代は	in junior high or high school
184	交叉させる(腕を)	Cross your arms
204	交叉させて重ねる(膝を)	cross one over the other
74	公衆浴場	a public bath
240	甲状腺に圧痛がある	You have thyroid tenderness
183	こうすると痛いですか	Does it hurt if I do this?
239	抗生剤	an antibiotic
295	抗体価	the antibody level of

INDEX

208	口内炎	a mouth ulcer
172	頚部硬直を診る	examine your neck for stiffness
166	肛門から出る	coming out of your bottom
206	こうやって～すると	When I lift your leg like this
197	号令をかける	I say
171	声を出す	say
314	呼吸器科の医者	pulmonologist (or: lung doctor)
178	呼吸する	breathe
213	呼吸センサー(一つは)	One is for your mouth and nose to record your breathing,
192	ここが痛む	Does this hurt?
33	ここが凹んでいる(乳の)	This part of my breast looks indented.
306	午後の診察は	Afternoon exams
75	心当たりはありますか(～という)	Do you have any idea if ~
142	心当たりはありませんか	Do you have any idea how
48	腰が痛い	My lower back hurts
237	腰の高さの棒	a bar at hip level
197	腰をかける(ベッドに)	sit up on the bed
102	腰を抜かす	Have you ever frozen up
301	腰を持つ	I'll grasp your lower back.
259	骨盤部のCT	a pelvic CT
97	コップ二杯(焼酎を)	two glasses of whisky or shochu
130	コップ半分	(a half) of a cup
300	ごと(シーツ)	together with the sheet
125	ことがありますか(聞こえる)	Do you ever hear wheezes
212	ことがある(違って見える)	can look different
143	今年初めて言われた	this is the first time you were told to
137	ことですか(～する)	do you mean ~
124	子供の頃に	when you were a child
242	後に(起きて数時間)	several hours after it developed
310	後に(数分)	After a couple of minutes
299	この後血液検査がある	After this, you'll have a blood exam
139	この種の動悸	this kind of palpitation
46	この徴候はあった(前から)	This started a while ago
221	この次に来る時	When you come next time
188	このように手を回す	twirl your hands around like this

67

197	このように手を組む	Hold both hands like this.
131	ご飯粒	rice or other food pieces
24	こぶができる(頭に)	have a bump on my head
105	こぼしたりしますか(口から)	Do you ever drool or drop food
105	こぼす(口から)	drool or drop food from your mouth
58	細かいぶつぶつ	a tiny red rash
30	ごみが入る(眼に)	have a speck in my eye
303	ゴムで腕を縛る	put a rubber band on your arm
167	こむらがえり	had a cramp in your calf
222	これ以上肥ると	If you gain more weight
207	これ位曲げる	like this
278	これ位を保つ	If you can keep to this
304	これで終った	Now we're finished.
312	これで終った	I think we're finished here
147	これまでもあった痛み	Have you had this pain before
114	ゴロゴロという低い音	low pitched rumble
53	転ぶ(自転車で)	fell off my bike
42	こわばる(手が)	My hands are stiff
139	今回初めてだ	is this the first time
277	今後	Beginning now
201	今度は左足で	Now try your left foot.
194	今度はへこませる	Now suck it in.
189	今度は眼を閉じて	This time, close your eyes

さ

129	細菌感染	a bacterial infection
159	最近だ(それは)	recent
81	最近どこかの	recently
9	最近のこと	recent things
46	最近は	now
299	採血室	the room for blood sampling
304	採血する (5ml)	take a 5 ml blood sample
304	採血する	draw blood
153	最後の生理	your last period
309	最後は〜となる	eventually just water will come out
231	最終診断には	to make a final diagnosis
168	最初にどこに	Where did you have your rash first?
221	最初の尿(朝起きて)	your first urine sample after you wake up

INDEX

148	最初は	at first
219	最長で8週間	8 weeks at most
295	最低一週間	at least 1 week
276	際に(次の受診の)	at your next visit
231	細胞の検査	An exam of cells
195	差がある(右と左で)	Is there any difference in pain on the left or right side?
195	差がある(痛みに)	Is there any difference in pain
273	下がる(熱が)	the fever goes away
311	先に呼ばれる	was called before me
197	下げる(脚を)	let your legs hang down
196	下げる(下着を)	take off your underwear
198	支える(身体を)	Support your body
44	ささくれだった竹	a bad bamboo splinter
44	刺さる(竹のとげが手に)	got a bad bamboo splinter in my hand
303	刺す(針を)	insert a needle
216	撮影体位	position in taking x-rays
246	雑音が(心臓に)	a heart murmur
307	寒い	feel cold
85	寒がりだ	often feel cold even if others do not
74	寒気がする	feel chilly
166	坐薬を使う	used a suppository
195	左右差がある(痛みに)	Is there any difference in pain on the left or right side?
69	触った感じという点で	in terms of touch
189	触る(指先で鼻先に)	touch your nose with your fingertip
133	参考までに	For reference
213	酸素の量	oxygen level
161	残尿感がある	feel a sensation called "constant urge to urinate"
130	3分の1	(a third)
	し	
300	シーツごと	together with the sheet
175	ジーッと見る	focus on
39	仕方がない(凝って)	nothing seems to help
48	仕方がない	there was nothing that could be done
152	しがち(下痢)	tend to have diarrhea

69

237	しがちだ (少なく)	tend to
138	しがちですか (どんな時に動悸)	When are you likely to have
166	痔が出る (肛門から)	had a hemorrhoid coming out of your bottom
269	しか認めない (4個以下しか)	there were less than 4 red blood cells
262	仕切られる	being partitioned or divided
103	仕事でコンピューターを使う	use a computer at work
104	仕事をする (コンピューターで)	working at the computer
316	自己負担分	Your self-pay ratio
38	しこりが触れる (腋の下に)	feel a lump in my armpit
268	示唆する所見 (石を)	sign suggesting kidney stones
238	歯周炎	gum disease
179	静かに息をする	breathe quietly
104	姿勢ですか (どんな)	What posture do you have
238	歯槽膿漏	perhaps an abscess
281	持続時間	the duration of the palpitation
112	持続する (頭痛が)	How long does the pain last
151	したい感じ (〜)	feel like 〜ing
212	次第で (条件設定)	depending on
212	従って	Thus
249	従って	Thus
301	下から抱える	lifting your knees from underneath
196	下着を下げる	take off your underwear
232	自宅でできる	you can do at home
310	したくなる (〜)	feel the need for having 〜
296	自宅療養	recuperation at home
251	下にした (胸膜を)	is trapezoidal, based on the pleura
146	下腹が痛む	Did the right upper (lower, left) side of your stomach hurt?
177	したままでいる (〜)	Keep your eyes closed
217	したら早めに (〜)	once you've finished
169	舌を出す	stick out your tongue
79	室温下に	at room temperature
277	しっかり管理する	make sure that
177	しっかり閉じる	closed tightly
139	失神する	blacked out

70

INDEX

208	湿疹はある	have pain or a rash
132	じっとしていても息切れする	Is it at rest
305	失敗した	This didn't work out.
295	指定する(会社が)	specified by the company
306	していただきます(〜)	we'd like you to see
45	していて(野球を)	playing baseball
140	していても(安静に)	even when you are resting
165	指摘される(血尿を)	pointed out to you that you have bloody urine
90	して下さい(〜)	May I see 〜
170	して下さい(〜)	Could you pull your lips
173	して下さい(〜)	Could you please 〜
175	して下さい(〜)	Can you focus on your nose?
187	して下さい(〜)	Can you do 〜
244	して下さい(〜しないで〜)	You should 〜. Don't 〜.
244	して下さい(〜)	You should place it under your tongue
279	して下さい(マスクを)	should wear a mask
279	して下さい(〜)	Be sure to wash your hands
289	して下さい(〜)	You should drink
295	して下さい(〜)	we need you to borrow
201	してみる(〜)	Try to stand on one foot.
46	しても(〜)	still there when I lie down
285	しても診断がつかない(〜を)	it remains undiagnosed after some exams
288	し通し(朝から〜)	you've been throwing up since this morning
101	自動車事故を起こす	had a car accident
264	しない限り(〜)	unless it causes
309	しないで下さい(〜)	you should not 〜
147	しばしばあった	very often
147	しばらくすると	after a while
79	しばらくの間	was there a time when you
266	しばらくの間	for a while
303	縛る(腕を)	put a rubber band on your arm
91	市販薬	over-the-counter drugs
228	耳鼻科(= 耳鼻科医)が	an ENT (ear, nose, throat) doctor
314	耳鼻科の医者	ENT doctor

71

316	自費になる (受診が)	the visit will be at your own expense
233	持病がある (他に)	have other chronic diseases
66	しびれがある (手足の)	have numbness in
190	しびれますか (手が)	Is there any numbness in your hand?
137	自分の脈	your pulse
259	脂肪組織	fat tissue
210	脂肪を調べる	lipids
222	しましょう (減量)	You should lose roughly 5 kg.
238	しましょう (禁煙)	you should quit smoking
254	しましょう (検査を)	Let me examine
278	しましょう (目安に)	We need to keep your urine output to
286	しましょう (〜に専念)	Let's focus on treatment.
288	しましょうか (点滴を)	some i.v. fluids would help
307	しましょうか (〜)	Would you like another blanket?
178	します (今から〜を)	Now I'd like to listen
310	します (浣腸)	Let me give you an enema.
301	しますね (〜)	Let me take your shoes off.
59	しみのようなものが出ている	have a kind of brownish age spot or liver spot
255	示している (それを)	as indicated by the fact that
140	示す (場所を手で)	show me the location
140	示す (指一本で場所を)	specify the location
72	しゃがんでいて	from sitting or crouching
249	写真 (CT)	CT picture
212	写真に (今日の)	in today's x-ray
214	写真は	The x-ray
215	シャワー	take a bath or shower
239	周囲に及ぶ	affecting the surrounding tissue
259	周囲の脂肪組織 (虫垂)	The surrounding fat tissue
241	収縮 (筋肉の)	muscle strain
101	集中力が欠けてきた	have trouble concentrating
141	週に何回位	How often do you have pain each week?
236	十分身体を休める	getting enough rest
278	十分だ (水分量は)	your water intake is fine
279	十分だ (水道水で)	Tap water is ok.
264	手術する	we don't operate
290	手術を考える	considering more invasive surgery

72

INDEX

303	手術を受けましたか(〜の)	Have you ever had surgery for ~
316	受診が自費になる	the visit will be at your own expense
230	受診した時点で	at the time of your visit
274	受診して下さい	come see me again
271	受診する(〜科を)	go see a dermatologist
312	受診する	Come and see me
211	受診当日の朝は	beginning the morning of your visit
276	受診の際に(次の)	at your next visit
316	受診の時に(月の最初の)	on the first visit of the month
305	酒精綿で	this cotton pad
238	出血する(歯茎から)	your gums bleed
297	守秘する(情報を)	maintain your information as confidential
231	腫瘍か	if this is an infection or a tumor
314	循環器科の医者	cardiologist
311	順番(私の)	my turn
228	紹介状を書く	I'll give you a referral.
306	紹介状を書く	made a referral
314	消化器科の医者	gastroenterologist (or: gastrointestinal doctor)
124	小学校時代は	in elementary school
272	消化のいい食べ物	bland food
290	衝撃波で	with ultrasonic waves
212	条件設定次第で	depending on the machine settings
247	上行大動脈に	in the ascending portion of the aorta
255	証拠だ(〜はその)	as indicated by the fact that ~
274	症状が	your symptoms
97	焼酎	whisky or shochu
259	状に(リング)	like a ring
314	小児科の医者	pediatrician
182	上半身を脱ぐ	take off your top
198	上半身	your upper body
90	情報提供紙(薬局の)	package insert from the pharmacy
297	情報(あなたの)	your information
75	賞味期限	its expiration date
280	除外する(可能性を)	rule out other possibilities
78	食あたり	food poisoning
98	食事の味付け	seasoning in food, like salt or spice

73

296	職場に復帰する	return to work
297	職場のだれにだったら	To whom in your office
297	職場の人が	someone from your office
10	食欲がない	I've lost my appetite. My appetite is poor.
229	所見(レントゲン写真の)	The x-ray findings
268	所見(～を示唆する)	sign suggesting kidney stones
239	所見から(喉の)	From the appearance of
247	所見がある(～という)	There is a finding called ~
299	処置室	treatment room
124	しょっちゅう休む	Were you frequently absent
89	処方する(薬を)	prescribe
271	処方する(痒み止めを)	prescribe some anti-itch medicine
317	処方箋	a prescription
242	処理した画像(～で)	image processed in a special way
205	知らせる(～に)	Tell me when
210	調べる(血液で～を)	examine the blood for ~
116	視力がいい	Is your eyesight good?
144	白っぽい	whitish
250	白っぽい領域	whitish area
259	白っぽく(より)	more whitish
7	白眼を出している	rolled back
248	心筋梗塞	a myocardial infarction or heart attack
56	人工関節	An artificial knee
178	深呼吸する	Take a deep breath in.
246	心雑音	a heart murmur
306	診察室の前で	in front of the consultation room
196	診察する(指で)	examine your anus using my finger
211	診察の前に	before you see the doctor
290	侵襲の大きい手術	more invasive surgery
314	心臓外科の医者	cardiac surgeon
268	腎臓の石	kidney stones
258	診断がつかない	we are still not sure of the diagnosis
285	診断がつかない	it remains undiagnosed
139	診断されましたか(何と)	What was the diagnosis
145	診断される(～と)	been diagnosed with ~
295	診断書	The medical certification

INDEX

296	診断書に	in this medical certificate
230	診断する (〜で)	Diabetes is diagnosed based on 〜
88	診断でしたか (どんな)	What diagnosis did your previous doctor give you?
218	診断できない (唾では)	can't be used for the diagnosis
302	身長	your height
178	心配いらない (あまり)	Things are probably o.k.
178	心配いらない (全く)	there's nothing to worry about
240	心配いらない	you don't have to worry
225	心配事がある時	When you're worried
256	心配しないで大丈夫	don't worry
227	心配するような所見はない	there's nothing to worry about
226	心配なら	If you're really worried
257	心房細動が (発作性の)	paroxysmal atrial fibrillation
95	蕁麻疹	hives
314	心療内科の医者	psychologist

す

230	随時に測った血糖	at the time of your visit even without fasting
279	水道の水	Tap water
272	水分 (多目の)	lots of fluids
278	水分量は十分だ	your water intake is fine
77	水分をとっている	drink something
138	睡眠時に	sleeping
110	睡眠中に	when you're asleep
224	睡眠薬	medicine for insomnia
245	吸う (息を)	inhale
238	吸う (歯茎を)	suck
307	吸う (鼻から酸素を)	inhale oxygen from your nose
309	数時間かけて	over several hours
236	数日間の潜伏期	a few days incubation period
180	ずーっと上に	all the way up
223	好き嫌いがある (食べ物に)	Are you particular about foods?
37	ズキズキ痛む (おできが)	throbs and hurts
65	ズキズキ脈打つ (痛みは)	Is the pain throbbing
75	過ぎた牛乳 (賞味期限が)	milk past its expiration date
151	すぐ後にまた (トイレに行った)	again soon after you go there

75

12	すくと(腹が)	when hungry
229	少ない(カリウムが)	potassium is low
196	すぐに終わる	I will finish soon.
219	すぐ分かる	know the result soon
288	少しずつでも飲めるなら	drink enough fluid, even little by little
289	少しずつ飲む	Drink a little bit
15	少し歪んでいる(顔が)	a bit crooked
249	スジ状の影	This black streak
275	進む(精密な検査に)	proceed to a more detailed exam
56	勧められた(人工関節を)	An artificial knee was recommended
226	勧める(薬を飲むことを)	I can recommend some medicine
248	勧める(検査を)	We recommend that
309	ずつ(一度に 200 ml)	one glass (200 ml) at a time
178	吸ったり吐いたりする	Breathe in slowly... Breathe out slowly...
159	ずっと前のことだ(それは)	Was it many years ago
300	ストレッチャーから	from the stretcher
53	砂や小石	some sand or dirt
62	腿にあざができる	got a purplish bruise on my thigh (calf)
289	スポーツ飲料	sports drinks
305	すみません	Excuse me.
309	済む(およそ 10 分で)	The exam itself is about 10 min.
53	擦りむく(膝を)	scratched my knees
258	する(検査を)	Let me do a blood test
220	するために(〜)	in order to prevent
237	すると〜が引き起こされる	which in turn leads to 〜
46	すると(〜)	when I lay down
255	すると軽くなる(〜)	improves when 〜
46	するのが常だった(〜)	It used to go away when I lay down
270	する人がいる(〜)	Some people have
296	すればいいですか(〜)	Should I 〜

せ

229	生化学検査(血液)	blood chemistry
215	生活をする(いつも通りの)	keep to your daily routine
317	請求される(調剤料が)	You will be charged
48	整形の医者	an orthopedic doctor
240	正常に戻す	bring it back to normal
314	精神科の医者	psychiatrist

INDEX

265	整腸剤	a pro-biotic
143	精密検査	a detailed exam
165	精密検査を受ける	have a thorough examination
135	整容	grooming
49	生理痛だ (ひどい)	have severe cramps
154	生理は不順だ	Is your period irregular
56	セカンドオピニオン	a second opinion on that
126	咳で目覚める	wake up coughing
224	咳止めがいい	you need some cough medicine
179	咳払いする	clear your throat
142	咳をする (大きな)	coughing violently
279	咳をする	has a cough
186	背筋を伸ばしてかける	sit up straight
250	石灰化陰影	a calcification shadow
244	舌下錠	a sublingual tablet
269	赤血球	red blood cells
272	摂氏38度	38 degrees Centigrade
251	接している (胸膜に)	is tangent to the pleura
266	絶食する	You won't be able to eat or drink
90	説明書 (薬の)	the explanation forms
220	説明書に	in the booklet
297	説明する (病状を)	explain your disease condition
220	説明は (詳しい)	Detailed explanations are
35	背中に痛みが走る	There's a sharp pain in my back
37	背中におできが	a pimple on my back
185	背中を診察する	examine your back
309	繊維の多い物	fibrous food
304	前回はどこから採血しましたか	Where did the nurse draw blood from before?
29	前頚部も腫れている	My throat is swollen, too.
309	前日の夜は	The night before
58	全身に出ている (発疹が)	have a tiny red rash all over
222	全身に問題が起きる	throughout your body
306	先生が	your doctor
124	喘息気味の	Were you asthmatic
128	全体が赤い (痰の)	uniformly reddish
286	専念する (治療に)	focus on treatment

77

236	潜伏期(数日間の)	a few days incubation period
125	喘鳴が聞こえる	hear wheezes
135	洗面	washing your face
228	専門だ(～は耳鼻科が)	one of their specialties is in treating ~
93	前立腺肥大症	prostatic hypertrophy

そ

258	造影CT検査	a contrast CT
247	造影剤を使って	with a contrast agent
215	そうしないと	otherwise
313	そうしないと～	Otherwise you will have to wait.
170	そう,そのように	Yes, like that.
287	鼠径ヘルニアだ	You have an inguinal hernia.
140	そこは痛む	Does it hurt
231	組織の検査	An exam of cells or tissue
261	組織検査	The tissue biopsy
261	組織診断	a tissue diagnosis
235	即効薬	quick cure or medicine
279	外から帰る	come indoors
305	その間	Meantime
220	その上で	Then
221	そのための容器	the container for that
232	そのための器械	a machine for that
165	その時、精密検査を	then
139	その時何と	What was the diagnosis then?
306	その前に	before then
46	そのままだ	it's still there
187	そのままでいる	do this for 10 seconds
203	そのままでいる(膝を立てて)	hold still
304	そのままでいる	don't move your arm
94	祖父母から子までの代の	from grandparents to children
303	それでは～して下さい	Then give me your other arm.
258	それでも～の時は	If we are still not sure of the diagnosis
72	それは～する時ですか	Is it when you suddenly stand up

た

124	体育をする	participated in sports
298	体温計	this thermometer
298	体温を測る	check your temperature

78

INDEX

251	台形のような形	The shape is trapezoidal
176	対光反射を診る	examine your light reflexes
234	退治する(ウィルスを)	kill viruses
302	体重	weight
95	帯状疱疹	herpes zoster infections
266	大丈夫～するから	don't worry, we'll give you
307	大丈夫	it's ok
236	大切だ(～が)	enough rest will be important
278	大切だ(～が)	You should not ～. This is important.
110	代だ(それは30)	Was it in your 30s?
260	大腸の憩室炎	colon diverticulitis
94	代の人(祖父母から子までの)	family members, from grandparents to children
287	大変な手術ではない	The surgery is not difficult
157	大便はどんな色ですか	What color is your stool?
133	平らな道を	on the level
7	倒れる(仰向けに)	fell down on his back
114	高い音(キーッという)	a high pitched squealing sound
277	高くなる(血圧が)	go up
302	高さに(臍の)	at the height of
277	高めだ(血圧が)	is rather high
238	だから止めましょう	so you should quit smoking
289	たくさん飲む(一度に)	drink too fast or too much at one time
136	だけ(～する時)	only when ～
233	だけだ(風邪を引いた)	you just have a common cold
233	だけで治る(～)	simply resting is enough to get well
169	出す(舌を)	stick out your tongue
286	出す(痰を)	bring up
303	出す(左腕を)	give me your left arm
189	出す(人差し指を)	pointing with your first finger
312	出す(窓口に)	take this folder to the receptionist
265	出す(悪いものを体の外に)	let bad things leave the body
195	叩く(軽く)	tap you lightly
101	ただのミスで起きる	a simple mistake
72	立ちくらみする	feel faint
310	経つと(数分)	After a couple of minutes
273	経てば(二日)	2 days after

79

204	立てる (膝を)	Pull your knees up
235	たとえ～だとしても	Even though you may ~
102	たとえば～	such as seeing things that aren't real
208	たとえば陰部や	such as your pubic area
72	たとえば、どんな時に	Give me an example of when
141	たとえば喉に通す	to other places such as your throat
110	たとえば旅行に行った時	For example, when you go on a trip
299	辿って行く (黄色い線を)	following the yellow line
101	たびに (目覚める)	every time you wake up
131	食べ物の一部	food pieces
75	食べる (悪い物を)	ate some bad food
268	溜まっている (便が)	there appears to be excessive fecal material
268	溜まる (液体が)	accumulation of fluid
134	ために (息苦しさの)	due to shortness of breath
232	ために (診断の)	To check this
224	ために (目覚める)	because of waking up
217	溜める (痰を)	collect your sputum
278	保つ (これ位を)	keep to this
123	だれかに (血縁者の)	Do any of your blood relatives have
279	だれでも咳をする人は	Everyone who has a cough
129	痰 (あなたの)	the phlegm you see
126	痰がからむ咳だ	you cough up phlegm
256	痰が出る (肺の病気になると)	Lung diseases sometimes produce sputum
264	胆管に落ち込む	falls into biliary duct
263	石が見つかる (胆嚢に)	A stone has been discovered in your gall bladder
290	胆石が	a gallstone
141	段々短くなっている (間隔は)	getting shorter and shorter
264	胆嚢炎	cholecystitis
263	胆嚢に	in your gall bladder
270	蛋白尿が出る	have protein in their urine
127	痰は出る	cough up phlegm (or: sputum)
130	痰はどれ位出ますか	How much phlegm do you produce
259	断面 (虫垂の)	the section of your appendix
218	痰を出す	cough up the sputum

80

INDEX

ち

253	小さい (角度が)	is smaller
317	近くの調剤薬局で	at your nearest dispensing pharmacy
81	近頃どこかの	recently
19	チカチカする感じ (眼が)	irritated
115	チカチカする (眼が)	feel a flushness or irritation in your eyes
234	違って (これと)	unlike this
212	違って見える	can look different
238	血が出る (歯茎から)	your gums bleed
57	力が入らない (足腰に)	My legs feel weak.
132	力仕事をした時	during physical activity
164	力を入れる (腹に)	push with your stomach
186	力を抜く (腕の)	let your arms relax
191	力を抜く (腹の)	relax your abdomen (or: stomach)
204	力を抜く	relax
310	力を抜く (お尻の)	Relax your bottom
303	チクッとします	You'll feel a slight pin prick.
249	乳首のレベルでの	at the level of the nipple
257	血の塊	clots
190	血の気が少なくなる	there's less circulation
94	血のつながりのある人	family members
59	茶色がかった	brownish
67	ちゃんと動く (手足は)	Are your arm and leg movements coordinated?
316	注意して下さい (〜ので)	Please note that ~
292	注意深く見る	pay attention when
124	中学時代は	in junior high or high school
92	注射で	drugs, either oral or by injection
306	昼食をとる	Please have lunch before then.
301	中心にして (お尻を)	with your hip as a pivot
258	虫垂炎	appendicitis
259	虫垂	your appendix
246	超音波検査	An ultrasound examination
258	超音波検査 (腹部)	abdominal ultrasound
263	超音波検査で	by ultrasound
190	徴候を検査する	check some signs

317	調剤薬局で	at your nearest dispensing pharmacy
317	調剤してもらう	fill it
317	調剤料	a drug and preparation fee
267	長時間我慢する (排尿を)	wait too long to urinate
266	腸閉塞だ	have a bowel obstruction
309	腸を空にする	empty your bowel
247	直後の部分 (枝分かれした)	portion of the aorta, which is right after it branches out
270	直後の尿 (起床)	urine right after they wake up
285	直接気管支鏡で	directly using a bronchoscope
84	ちょっとした腹痛	slight stomach ache
235	治療法	cure
124	治療を必要とする	require any treatment
234	鎮痛剤	a painkiller

つ

48	椎間板ヘルニア	a slipped disc
263	追跡する	be followed up
158	ついてだが (頻尿に)	Regarding frequent urination
313	通常の診療	regular office visits
47	通知を受ける (～するよう)	was told to get ~
265	使う (下痢止めを)	take anti-diarrheal medicines
295	使う (診断書用紙を)	use our form
247	使って (造影剤を)	with a contrast agent
237	つかまって (棒に)	hold on to a bar
301	つかまる (私に)	hold on to me
13	疲れが抜けない	feel tired
180	突き出す (胸の右側を)	push the right side of your chest out
301	次に身体を回す	Next, I'll turn you
281	次に動悸を感じたら	When you have palpitations next time
316	月の最初の受診の時に	on the first visit of the month
311	次の次だ (順番は)	Your turn is the one after next.
211	次は (この)	Next time
199	次はつま先で立つ	then stand on your toes
45	つき指をする	jammed my finger
198	つく (ベッドに両膝を)	Put both knees on the bed
213	付け方は (センサーの)	how to attach the sensors
198	付けて (手を間仕切りに)	touching the partition with both hands

INDEX

248	付ける (記録器を身体に)	wear a small monitor
213	付けるセンサー (身体に)	sensors attached to your body
308	都合がいいですか (いつが)	When would be convenient for you?
211	続ける (薬を)	continue taking your usual medicines
32	つっかえる (食べ物が)	have difficulty swallowing
274	続く (症状が)	your symptoms persist
84	続く病気 (一週間以上)	any illness lasting more than a week
206	突っ張る (腿の後ろが)	feel tense
216	つながる (見落としに)	can lead to missing of
46	常だった (~するのが)	It used to go away when I lay down
218	唾では診断できない	Saliva can't be used for the diagnosis
144	唾のように	like saliva
199	つま先で立つ	stand on your toes
200	つま先をくっつけて (左右の踵と)	with heels and toes touching each other
142	つまづいて転ぶ	tripping and falling down
264	詰まらせる (管を)	stops it up
257	詰まる (血管に)	blocking the vessels
110	詰まる (鼻が)	Does your nose become stuffy?
69	冷たさという点で	coolness
34	つゆが出る (乳首から)	There's a discharge from my nipple.
249	強い (疑いが)	we strongly suspect
112	強い光	bright lights
238	強く吸う (歯茎を)	suck strongly
234	強くする (打ち勝つ力を)	building up your strength
112	強くなる (痛みが)	make the pain worse
291	強くなる (痛みが)	make your pain worse
140	強さ (痛みの)	the intensity of the pain
240	つれて (治るに)	as inflammation goes down

て

7	手足が痙攣する	His arms and legs were cramping.
66	手足のしびれ	numbness in your hands or legs
236	手洗い	washing hands
263	定期的に	regularly
295	提出期限はいつですか	When is the due date of submission?
222	程度 (5キロ)	roughly 5 kg
73	程度が同じ (起きてから今まで)	Is it about the same since it started

83

213	テープで貼りつける	with tape
264	摘出する	take it out
62	できる(あざが)	got a purplish bruise
261	できる(外来で)	can be done in the out-patient clinic
214	できる(写真は)	The x-ray will be ready
37	できる(背中におできが)	have a pimple on my back
169	できるだけ前に出す	stick out your tongue as far as possible
181	できるだけ大きく吸う	Take a deep breath in, as far as you can go.
181	できるだけ速く	as fast as possible
276	できれば～して下さい	If you can, check
262	凸凹に見える(中が)	looks irregular inside
244	です(～)	Note that ~
259	です(これは骨盤部のCT)	This is a pelvic CT.
238	ですから止めましょう	so you should quit smoking
124	ですね(～をしていたの)	I understand ~
24	手すりにぶつける(頭を)	hit my head on the handrail
46	出て来る(立つと)	stick out when I stand up
292	出て来ないか見る(石が)	see a stone come out
140	手で示す	using your hand
187	手のひらを上にする	Turn your palms up
283	で増える(心筋梗塞)	with myocardial infarction
131	出る(血痰は)	Did bloody sputum come out
166	出る(肛門から)	coming out of your bottom
247	出る(大動脈が心臓から)	it branches out from the heart
130	出る(痰が)	you produce
42	手を握る時に	when I make a fist
301	手を回して(私の肩に)	with your arms around my shoulders
168	電気が走るような痛み	a tingling pain like an electric jolt
7	天井を向く(眼は)	His eyes were focused on the ceiling
128	点状に赤い	spotty with tiny red spots
133	電柱	electrical poles
69	点で(～という)	in terms of ~
266	点滴で	by i.v.
288	点滴をしましょうか	some i.v. fluids would help
313	電話する(前もって)	call ahead
297	電話で説明する	talk about the patients' disease condition by phone

84

INDEX

と

297	問い合わせて来る	asks
158	トイレに起きる	wake up to go to bathroom
101	トイレに立つ	you go to the bathroom
297	同意書 (患者の)	a consent form for the patient
137	動悸 (あなたの言う)	When you say "palpitation"
138	動悸する	have palpitations
313	当日受診の場合でも	Even if it's for a same day visit
309	当日の朝	the morning of the exam
63	どうしましたか	How are you doing? etc.
213	同席する (お家の方が)	if a family member could be with you
81	どうですか (あなたの学校は)	How about your school?
95	どうですか (花粉症は)	How about hay fever
122	どうですか (洟の硬さは)	What is the consistency of any nasal discharge?
129	透明な痰	clear phlegm
76	同僚	coworkers
110	同僚	your coworker
174	遠くの方を見る	look straight ahead
141	通す (痛みは他の所に)	Does the chest pain travel to other places
309	溶かす (2 リットルの水に)	dissolve
244	溶かす (自然に)	let it dissolve
71	時ですか (〜するのは〜する)	When 〜 , is it when 〜 ?
72	時ですか (それは〜する)	Is it when you suddenly stand up
106	時に痛い (飲み込む)	Does it hurt to swallow?
163	途切れる (尿が)	have interrupted urine flow, or urine flow that starts and stops
242	特殊な方法で	in a special way
140	特定する (場所を)	specify the location
256	特に労作時に	especially when exercising
252	とげ (ウニの)	sea urchin spines
44	とげ (竹の)	a bad bamboo splinter
108	どこが痛みますか (喉の)	Where in the throat does it hurt?
115	どこが痛みますか (頭の)	Where in your head does it hurt?
140	どこが痛みますか (胸の)	Where does it hurt in your chest?
146	どこが痛いですか (腹の)	Where did it hurt in your stomach?

63	どこが具合が悪いですか	How are you feeling? etc.
208	どこかに (口以外の)	elsewhere other than your mouth
142	どこかにぶっつける (胸を)	hitting your chest on something
81	どこかの学校が	a school
304	どこから採りましたか	Where did the nurse draw blood from
48	年のせいで仕方がない	it was age related
177	閉じる (眼を)	Keep your eyes closed
64	年をとると	When people grow older
163	途中で (排尿の)	When you are urinating
224	途中で目覚める	waking up often during the night
113	どちらか一方がより良く~	is one better than the other
234	特効薬がある (インフルエンザには)	For the flu, we do have special medicine.
234	特効薬はない	have no medicine to kill viruses
193	どっちが痛いですか	Does it hurt more when I ~ or when I ~?
196	届く範囲に (指の)	within the reach of my finger
106	どの辺りが (喉の)	Where in your throat
238	とのことから (血が出る)	You said your gums bleed
288	とのことなので (~)	You said you've been ~
219	塗抹検査	smear examination
284	塗抹検査で	in a sputum smear examination
271	とりあえず	for now
278	摂り過ぎる (水分を)	drink too much water or fluids
290	取り出す (石を)	take it out
272	摂る (多目の水分を)	drink lots of fluids
304	採る	draw blood
285	採る (細胞や組織を)	pick cells or tissue
214	とる (心電図を)	take an electrocardiogram
214	撮る (胸のX線写真を)	take a chest x-ray
284	とる (防止措置を)	practice infection prevention
282	撮る (レントゲン写真を)	take x-rays
85	どれ位ですか (平熱は)	What is your normal body temperature?
96	どれ位の頻度で	How often
132	どれ位でなくなりますか (息切れは)	How long does your shortness of breath last
133	どれくらい歩けますか	How long can you walk
122	ドロッとしている	Thick like mucus

INDEX

253	鈍角だ	(obtuse) angle
127	どんな色ですか	What color is it?
144	どんな色ですか(それは)	What was the color
157	どんな色ですか(大便は)	What color is your stool?
13	どんなことをしても	no matter what I do
104	どんな姿勢ですか	What posture do you have
88	どんな診断でしたか	What diagnosis did your previous doctor give you?
64	どんな時に同じことを言いましたか	when she has repeated herself
132	どんな時に	When
138	どんな時に	When
234	頓服の鎮痛剤を飲む	take a painkiller as needed
265	頓服の痛み止め	a painkiller to be taken as needed

な

306	内科診察の後	After an examination by the internist
314	内科の医者	internist
91	ないですか(飲んでいる薬は)	Are you taking any drugs
252	内部に空洞も見える	can also see the cavity inside
314	内分泌科の医者	endocrinologist
102	無いはずの物が見える	seeing things that aren't real
86	治りますか(何日で)	how long does it typically last
233	治る(安静だけで)	get well
240	治る(炎症が)	inflammation goes down
262	中が凸凹に見える	looks irregular inside
51	長く歩くと	when I walk a long way
252	中に空洞も見える	can also see the cavity inside
249	中に見える影(気管支が)	the shadow with bronchial tubes seen inside
17	流れる(よだれが)	drool from one side of my mouth
132	なくなる(息切れは)	does your shortness of breath last
202	なぞり下ろす(踵を足首まで)	slide your heel down to the ankle
205	なったら(〜しなく)	when you cannot sense the vibration any more
240	なっている(過剰に)	have excessive thyroid hormone
111	など(むち打ち症)	such as whiplash
282	斜めから撮る	diagonally

87

75	何か悪い物	some bad food
211	何も食べずに	you should not eat anything
144	何を吐いたのですか	What kind of stuff did you throw up?
21	鍋でもかぶっている感じだ	feels heavy
79	生で食べる	eat raw oysters
78	生ものによる	by eating raw food (or: from raw food)
80	生焼きだ(焼き鳥が)	was not cooked well
147	波がなく続く痛み	constant, dull pain
25	涙が多い	My eyes water.
25	涙眼だ	My eyes water.
141	舐める(薬を)	take the medicine
315	並ぶ(一列に)	form a line
255	なる(〜位から〜位に)	going from lying down to sitting up
141	何回位感じますか	How often do you have pain
101	何回目覚めますか	How often do you wake up
8	何回も聞き返す	asks the same things repeatedly
101	何時間位寝ますか	How long do you sleep
103	何時間〜しますか(一日)	How long during the day do you use a computer
132	何時間もかかる	as long as few hours
48	何とか良くならないか	still hope something's possible
209	何の手術の痕ですか	What kind of surgery was that for?
99	何本吸いますか(一日、およそ)	About how many cigarettes do you smoke per day?

に

179	二回咳払いする	clear your throat twice
303	握る(手を軽く)	make a light fist
42	握る時に(手を)	when I make a fist
129	濁った黄色や緑色の痰	an opaque yellowish or greenish phlegm
162	濁っている(尿が)	Is your urine cloudy or clear?
47	二次検診	a second medical check
135	日常生活動作で	when doing daily activities
153	日に(11月16)	on November 16
288	日分の〜薬(二)	two days worth of 〜 medicine
224	日中疲れ不足なら	If you feel tired during the day
41	にぶい(手の感覚が)	There's a dull or numb sensation in my hand.

88

INDEX

95	入院するような病気	disease that required hospitalization
261	入院する	be admitted to the hospital
266	入院して	will require hospitalization
287	入院費用	cost for both outpatient and inpatient care
303	乳がん (片方の)	breast cancer on one side
135	入浴	having a bath
162	尿が濁っている	Is your urine cloudy or clear?
268	尿管の石	kidney stones
164	尿漏れはある	have urine leakage
278	尿量	your urine output
153	妊娠の可能性はある	Do you think you might be pregnant?

ぬ

266	抜く (ガスを)	relieve your gas
182	脱ぐ (上半身を)	take off your top
44	抜く (とげを)	pulled it out

ね

300	ね (~します)	We have to move you
102	寝入りばなに	when falling asleep
71	寝返りする時	when you roll over in bed
184	猫背になる	curl up into a ball
260	熱が出る病気	diseases with fever
224	寝つきがいい	you may fall asleep quickly
272	熱さまし	a fever reducing medicine
272	熱のある時は	If you get a fever
22	熱をもっている (おでこが)	feels hot
110	寝ている時に	when you're asleep
101	寝てから起きるまで	in the middle of the night
46	寝てもそのまま	still there when I lie down
224	寝不足だ (日中)	feel tired during the day
101	眠くなる	become sleepy
102	眠っていて	when you are asleep
224	眠れないのであれば	If you wake up
202	寝る (仰向けに)	lie down on your back
191	寝る (ベッドに)	Lie back on the bed
122	粘液のように	like mucus
157	粘液のようなもの	what looks like a sticky fluid

89

55	捻挫する(足首を)	sprained it
47	年に一度の健診の	an annual health checkup
314	脳外科の医者	brain surgeon
257	脳梗塞を起こす	causing a stroke
241	脳出血	in your brain, such as bleeding
262	嚢胞性陰影	cystic shadow
239	膿瘍の可能性がある	an abscess is possible
44	残っている(とげが中に)	there's some left
53	残っている(小石が)	dirt is left inside
161	残っている(尿が)	you still need to urinate
172	載せる(頭を私の手に)	Place your head on my hand.
301	載せる(お尻をベッドに)	Place your hip on the bed.
202	載せる(踵を反対側の脚の膝に)	place your heel on the other leg's knee
186	載せる(手を膝に)	Put both hands on your knees.
265	望ましい(〜するのが)	it's best to let bad things leave
70	乗っている(船に)	like riding in a boat
291	ので(痛みが強くなる)	as they make your pain worse
106	喉のどの辺りが	Where in your throat
213	喉仏	your Adam's apple
29	喉も腫れている	My throat is swollen, too.
186	伸ばしてかける(背筋を)	sit up straight
187	伸ばす(腕を)	extend your arms
136	上り坂を上る	climbing up a hill
92	飲み薬で	drugs, either oral or by injection
244	飲み込む	swallow it directly
106	飲み込む時(つばを)	Does it hurt to swallow?
90	飲む(薬を)	What medication are you taking?
91	飲む(薬を)	Are you taking any drugs

は

225	場合は(その)	In that case
270	場合は(その)	In that case
273	場合は(〜の)	With flu
249	肺炎の疑いが濃い	we strongly suspect pneumonia
201	はい、下ろして下さい	Ok, good.
301	はい、下ろして下さい	Now lower your head. Good.
196	はい、終わった	Now it's done.

90

INDEX

129	ばい菌による炎症	a bacterial infection
267	ばい菌を洗い流す	wash out the bacteria
135	排泄	going to the toilet
144	吐いたのですか(何を)	What kind of stuff did you throw up?
55	履いていて(高い靴を)	wearing high heels
156	排尿する	urinate
160	排尿する	urinate
253	肺の方から	from the lung towards the pleura
156	排便する	have a bowel movement
310	排便する(我慢してから)	before having a bowel movement
219	培養検査	culture
230	測る(血糖を)	take a measurement
213	測る(酸素の量を)	for measuring the oxygen level
281	測る(持続時間を)	record the duration
276	測る(体温を)	check your temperature
298	測る(体温を)	check your temperature
247	剥がれる(壁と壁の間が)	three layers of the arterial wall start to peel apart
257	剥がれる(血の塊が)	breaking loose of clots
66	吐き気がありますか	any nausea
288	吐き気止め	anti-nausea medicine
220	吐き気を抑える	prevent coughing and gagging
307	吐きたい時は	If you need to throw up
245	吐く(息を)	exhale
307	吐く(ここに)	you can do it here
238	歯茎から血が出る	your gums bleed
140	漠然とした範囲の痛み	a rather vague (or: dull) pain
65	拍動する(痛みは)	Is the pain throbbing
298	はさむ(体温計を腋の下に)	place this thermometer in your armpit
95	はしか	measles
40	箸でつかもうとして	from my chopsticks
153	始まる(生理が)	My period started
306	始まる(診察は3時に)	Afternoon exams begin at 3.
165	初めて指摘される	When was it first pointed out
139	初めてだ(今回)	is this the first time
160	始めの方で(排尿の)	when you start urinating
11	始める(薬を飲み)	I began taking drugs (or: medication) for

91

140	場所 (痛む)	the location of the pain
35	走る (背中に痛みが)	There's a sharp pain in my back
304	外す (ゴムを)	release the band
172	外す (枕を)	remove the pillow
253	発育する (肺の方から胸膜に向かって)	grows from the lung towards the pleura
6	はっきりしない (意識が)	My father seems alert but a bit confused.
21	はっきりしない (頭が)	My head's not clear.
252	はっきりした (境界が)	its edges are sharply defined
118	はっきりと見える (眼は)	Is your eyesight OK?
236	発症する	Flu develops
1	ぱっとしない (気分が)	don't feel well
110	鼻が詰まる	Does your nose become stuffy?
119	洟が出ますか	Do you have any nasal discharge
107	洟が喉の後ろを伝って	running down the back of my throat
307	鼻から酸素を吸う	inhale oxygen from your nose
175	鼻先を	nose
68	話をすることが難しい	have difficulty making conversation
193	離す時 (手を)	when I let up
121	鼻血が出る	Do you ever get nose bleeds
120	鼻づまり	Any nasal obstruction
102	ばなに (寝入り)	when falling asleep
177	鼻の孔	your nostrils
121	洟の色	the color of any nasal discharge
122	洟の硬さ	the consistency of any nasal discharge
213	鼻の下に	under your nose
120	鼻は詰まる	Does your nose get clogged shut?
119	鼻水が出る	a runny nose
121	鼻をかむと	when you blow your nose
181	速く息を吐く (できるだけ)	blow out as fast as possible
178	速く呼吸する (少し)	breathe a little faster
235	速く治す治療法	quick cure
137	速くなること (脈が)	a fast pulse
217	早めに (~したら)	once you've finished
316	払い戻す	refund the money
12	腹がすくと	when hungry
249	腹側 (こっちが)	This is the abdominal side.

INDEX

144	腹の具合はいい	Does your stomach now feel all right?
191	腹の力を抜く	relax your abdomen (or: stomach)
196	腹の方に持ち上げる(両膝を)	move them closer to your stomach
146	腹の真ん中が痛む	Did it hurt in the middle of your stomach
146	腹の右上が痛む	Did the right upper (lower, left) side of your stomach hurt?
268	腹のレントゲン写真	an abdominal x-ray image
207	腹這いになる	Turn back over on your stomach
150	腹は弱い	have a weak stomach
149	バリウムでする(胃の検査を)	have a barium contrast x-ray, or a gastric camera exam for stomach checkup
213	貼り付ける(センサーを)	be attached around your Adam's apple
303	針を刺す	insert a needle
29	腫れている(まぶたが)	My eyelid is swollen.
238	歯を磨く	brush your teeth
170	歯を見せるように	showing your teeth
315	番号順に	in numeric order
96	晩酌する	drink alcohol with dinner
61	絆創膏にかぶれる	had a funny skin reaction to the Band-Aid
202	反対側の脚の膝に載せる	place your heel on the other leg's knee
231	判断がつかない(感染症か)	We can't determine if
247	判断する(解離が~の原因と)	this is the likely cause of ~
223	半年で	over the past 6 months
130	半分(コップ)	(a half) of a cup

ひ

291	控える(脂っこい物を)	avoid fatty foods
259	皮下脂肪	subcutaneous fat
237	引き起こされる(すると~が)	which in turn leads to muscle weakness
260	引き起こされる(病気が)	This disease is caused by
114	低い音(ゴロゴロという)	low pitched rumble
186	膝に載せる(手を)	Put both hands on your knees.
202	膝に載せる(踵を)	place your heel on the other leg's knee
222	膝の関節	knee joints
237	膝の曲げ伸ばしをする	squat down and up
53	膝を擦りむく	scratched my knees
203	膝を立てる	raise your knees up

204	膝を立てる	Pull your knees up
53	肘を擦りむく	scratched my knees and elbows
143	引っかかる(胸のレントゲンが)	An abnormal chest x-ray was found
102	びっくりする	being surprised
46	ひっこむ(横になると)	go away when I lay down
252	引っ張られる	are pulled towards it
197	引っ張る(手を両側に)	pull on them
261	必要がある(組織診断をする)	requires a tissue diagnosis
261	必要がある(入院する)	need to be admitted to the hospital
263	必要がある(追跡する)	This should be followed up
285	必要がある(組織を採る)	we need to pick cells
231	必要だ(組織の検査が)	will be needed to make
295	必要だ(最低一週間)	We need at least 1 week
124	必要とする(治療を)	require any treatment
295	必要とする項目(〜が)	the requirement by 〜
248	否定する(狭心症を)	rule out angina on effort
254	否定する(結核を)	rule out tuberculosis
234	ひどい(頭痛が)	If your headache is bad
49	ひどい生理痛だ	have severe cramps
250	ひと際白い影	a markedly white shadow
8	ひどくなる(〜が)	〜 has become worse
189	人差し指	your first finger
219	一つは〜もう一つは〜	One way is called 〜. Another is called 〜.
176	瞳の大きさ	the size of your pupils
314	泌尿器科の医者	urologist
14	微熱がある	have a low grade fever
55	ひねる(足首を)	twisted my ankle
35	ひねると(身体を)	when I twist
303	響く(痛みが指先に)	Does the pain travel to your fingertips?
314	皮膚科の医者	dermatologist
12	冷や汗が出る	break into a cold sweat
222	標準	normal
242	描出されている	visible
297	病状(あなたの)	your disease condition
269	病的と見なさない	we don't think this is caused by disease
304	開く(手を)	Open your fist.
168	平べったい	Is it flat

94

INDEX

109	ヒリヒリする感じだ(喉は)	Does your throat feel like it's burning
168	ピリピリする痛み	a tingling pain
43	昼前には	by noon
47	貧血がある	the blood was anemic
96	頻度で(どれ位の)	How often
158	頻尿	frequent urination
119	頻繁に出る(くしゃみが)	sneeze often
225	頻脈になる	your heart rate can go up

ふ

312	ファイルを(この)	this folder
225	不安な時	anxious
95	風疹	rubella
283	増えているか検査する	check the level of
225	増える(脈が)	your heart rate can go up
100	ふかす(タバコは)	inhale tobacco smoke shallowly
302	腹囲	waist size
290	腹腔鏡で	laparoscopically
92	副作用が出る(薬で)	Have you had any reactions to drugs
240	副腎皮質ホルモン	a steroid
314	腹部外科の医者	abdominal surgeon
91	含めて(市販薬を)	including over-the-counter drugs
222	含めて(膝の関節を)	including knee joints
169	膨らませる(ほっぺを)	puff out your cheeks
177	膨らませる(鼻の孔を)	Flare your nostrils.
194	膨らませる(腹を)	Push your stomach out.
46	膨らんでいる(脚の付け根が)	have a bulge in my groin
43	節々が痛む	the joint soreness
154	不順だ(生理は)	Is your period irregular
314	婦人科の医者	gynecologist (or: OB/GYN doctor)
306	婦人科を受診する	see an OB-GYN doctor
26	二つに見える	I see double.
116	二つに見える(物が)	have double vision
150	普段から〜しがち	tend to have soft stools
101	普段何時間位寝ますか	How long do you sleep usually?
86	普段は何日で治りますか	how long does it typically last
264	普通だ(手術しないのが)	usually we don't operate
216	普通の写真では	In one conventional image

275	普通の写真で	on the x-ray
296	復帰する(職場に)	return to work
24	ぶつける(頭を手すりに)	hit my head on the handrail
142	ぶつける(胸をどこかに)	hitting your chest on something
283	物質(血液中に増える)	a substance that increases in the blood
259	太さは1センチだ	It's one centimeter thick.
220	太さは鉛筆と同じ	Its diameter is
222	肥っている	You are overweight
222	肥ると(これ以上)	If you gain more weight
70	船に乗っている	like riding in a boat
247	部分	portion of the aorta
249	部分は(この)	This area looks whiter
24	踏み外す(階段を)	tripped on some stairs
224	不眠なのであれば	If you wake up
147	ぶり返す(痛みが)	comes back again
274	ぶり返す(症状が)	get better but then come back
74	振える(体が)	shiver
205	振えを感じる	sense the vibration
38	触れる(しこりが)	feel a lump
54	ブロックが(壁から)	Some bricks from a wall fell on me
268	糞塊(大量の)	excessive fecal material
309	分で終わる(およそ10)	The exam itself is about 10 min.
288	分の〜薬(二日)	two days worth of 〜 medicine
309	粉末の下剤	this powdered laxative
214	分もあればできる(〜)	The x-ray will be ready within twenty minutes.

へ

268	閉塞した腸に	in the obstructed bowel
85	平熱は	your normal body temperature
133	ペースで(あなたの)	at your own pace
194	へこませる(腹を)	suck it in
33	凹んでいる(ここが)	looks indented
146	臍の下が痛む	Did it hurt in the middle of your stomach (under your bellybutton)?
302	臍の高さに	at the height of your bellybutton
300	ベッドに移りますね	from the stretcher to the bed
87	別の医者に	another doctor

INDEX

87	別の病院に	to another hospital
236	経て(潜伏期を)	over a few days incubation period
246	弁(心臓の)	the heart valves
268	便(大量の)	excessive fecal material (or: stool)
155	便意がある	feel like having a bowel movement
293	返却する	return the monitor
316	返金する	We will refund the money
243	片頭痛	Migraine headache
280	片頭痛の発作は	Migraine attacks
47	便潜血検査	the stool blood test
155	便通がある	have a bowel movement (or: BM)
239	扁桃腺	your tonsil
213	弁当箱位の大きさだ	is the size of a bento-box
157	便はどんな色ですか	What color is your stool?
152	便秘する	have diarrhea or constipation
268	便秘だ(原因は)	Constipation may then be a cause

ほ

267	膀胱炎だ	have a urinary bladder infection
314	放射線科の医者	radiologist
165	放置していて構わない	this is nothing to worry about
219	方法で(二通りの)	in two ways
242	方法で(特殊な)	in a special way
2	ボーッとしている	don't feel alert
76	他のだれかに	Is there anyone else
141	他の所に通す(痛みは)	travel to other places
260	他の病気(熱が出る)	other diseases with fever
249	他より白い	looks whiter than other area
79	保管する(かきを)	keep them in a refrigerator
297	保険会社の人	a person from the insurance company
56	欲しい(セカンドオピニオンが)	want a second opinion on that
295	母子健康手帳	your mother-child notebook
287	保証はない(100％安全という)	nothing is 100% guaranteed
220	細い(胃カメラより)	thinner than a gastric camera
304	細い(血管が)	your vessels are thin
257	発作性の心房細動が	paroxysmal atrial fibrillation
58	発疹が	a tiny red rash
169	ほっぺを膨らませる	puff out your cheeks

97

58	ぽつぽつが	a tiny red rash
170	微笑むように	like you're smiling
261	ポリープがある	have a polyp
216	ほんのわずかな変化	the slightest change of
27	ぼんやりしか見えない	My vision is blurry.

ま

213	マイクロホン(喉)	a small throat microphone
31	毎年今頃	Every year at this time
201	前足の踵	the heel of the front one
136	前かがみになる	bend forward
184	前で交叉させる(腕を)	Cross your arms in front of you
290	前に(〜を考える)	before considering 〜
211	前に(診察の)	before you see the doctor
309	前に(大腸カメラの)	Before the colonoscopy
187	前に(まっすぐ)	straight ahead
88	前の医者	your previous doctor
309	前の日の夜は	The night before
108	前の方が(喉の)	front of the throat
185	前向きに戻る	turn around and face me again
313	前もって電話する	call ahead
15	曲がっている(顔が)	My face feels a bit crooked.
302	巻き尺を当てて測る	measure it by using a tape measure
301	枕を入れる	put a pillow under your head
207	曲げる(脚を)	Bend your legs
190	曲げる(腕を)	flex your arm
184	曲げる(首を前に)	tuck your chin to your chest
60	負ける(化粧品に)	had an allergic reaction to this cosmetic
160	まさに終わろうとする時	when you are about to finish
198	間仕切りに向く	facing the partition
157	混じっている(ようなものは)	contain what looks like
131	混じる(痰に食物の一部が)	Did your bloody sputum contain
127	混じる(血が)	Does it contain blood?
295	麻疹の抗体価	the antibody level of measles
201	先ず〜、今度は〜	First 〜. Now 〜.
314	麻酔科の医者	anesthesiologist
220	麻酔をする(喉に)	give you an anesthetic in your throat
279	マスクをする	wear a mask

98

INDEX

301	先ずつかまる	First, hold on to me
311	まだですか (順番は)	Is my turn yet?
299	待合室	waiting room
312	待つ (予約日まで)	wait for your next appointment
67	まっすぐ歩く	walk straight
187	まっすぐ前に伸ばす	extend your arms straight ahead
174	まっすぐ見る	look straight
178	全く心配いらない	there's nothing to worry about
311	待っている (一時間)	have been waiting for 1 hour
180	まで (耳にくっつく)	until it touches your ear
306	窓口で (受け付け)	at the reception window
29	まぶたが腫れている	My eyelid is swollen.
207	ままでいる (この)	hold still
301	回して (私の肩に手を)	with your arms around my shoulders
301	回す (身体を)	I'll turn you
188	回す (手を)	twirl your hands around
252	まわりの血管 (陰影の)	vessels around this shadow
70	回る (壁が)	walls are rotating

み

216	見失う (異常陰影を)	missing of abnormal shadows
27	見えない (ぼんやりしか)	My vision is blurry.
212	見えない (異常陰影が)	we don't see any abnormal shadows
28	見えなくなる (右眼が)	I went blind on the right side
304	見えにくい (血管が)	your vessels are thin and difficult to find
242	見える (血管が)	visible
212	見える (違って)	can look different
262	見える (中が凸凹に)	looks irregular inside
118	見える (眼ははっきりと)	Is your eyesight OK?
26	見える (二つに)	I see double.
249	見える (より白く)	looks whiter
259	見える (リング状に)	looks like a ring
216	見落とす (異常陰影を)	missing of abnormal shadows
180	右側を (胸の)	right side of your chest
69	右と左で差がある	Is there any difference in your sensations on the left or right side
260	右の下腹部が痛む病気	diseases with fever and right-side lower stomach pain

113	右左で同じように聞こえる	hear equally well in both ears
122	水っぽい	watery
101	ミスで起きる	was it a simple mistake
211	水で飲む (薬を)	taking your usual medicines with water
309	水のような便	You will have watery diarrhea
168	水膨れ	blisters
95	水疱瘡	chicken pox
97	水割り (焼酎の)	whisky or shochu with water
90	見せて下さい	May I see
276	見せて下さい (受診の際に)	show me the results at your next visit
148	みぞおち辺りが	around the pit of your stomach
295	満たす (必要項目を)	fulfill
88	見たてをする	What diagnosis did your previous doctor give you?
137	乱れること (脈が)	irregular pulse
263	見つかる (石が)	A stone has been discovered in
175	見つめる (鼻先を)	focus on your nose
271	診てもらう (皮膚科で)	go see your dermatologist
196	認めない (異常を)	didn't recognize any abnormal area
121	緑がかった	greenish
269	見なさない (病的と)	we don't think this is caused by disease
114	耳鳴りがする	Do you have any ringing in your ears?
65	脈打つ (痛みは)	Is the pain throbbing
137	脈が速くなること	do you mean a fast pulse
225	脈が増える	your heart rate can go up
281	脈の数を数える	count your pulse
137	脈をみる (自分の)	feel your pulse
190	脈をみる (後ろから)	check your pulse from behind
242	見る (〜の影響を)	we can see the effects of a stroke
172	診る (首の硬さを)	examine your neck for stiffness
175	見る (じーっと)	focus on my fingertip
176	診る (対光反射を)	examine your light reflexes
191	診る (腹を)	check your abdomen
281	みる (乱れていないかどうかを)	check if your pulse is regular

む

9	昔のこと	things of the past
196	向って (壁に)	facing the wall

INDEX

252 向かって (陰影に)	towards it
198 向く (間仕切りに)	facing the partition
174 向く (私の方にまっすぐ)	look straight at me
185 向く (私の方を)	face me
57 むくむ (脚が)	My legs are swollen.
117 むくんでいる (顔が)	your face looks puffy
190 向ける (顔を左に)	Turn your head to the left.
118 虫が飛ぶ症状 (眼の前で小さな)	symptom such as eye floaters
68 難しい (話をすることが)	have difficulty making conversation
31 ムズムズする (鼻が)	my eyes and nose are itchy
111 むち打ち症	whiplash
137 胸苦しさ	feel chest tightness
141 胸の痛み	the chest pain
143 胸のレントゲン	chest x-ray
145 胸焼けがある	heartburn or a burning sensation when you burp
62 紫色の	purplish
235 無理だ (申し出は)	There is no ~ that I can

め

252 明瞭な (境界が)	its edges are sharply defined
116 眼鏡が合っている	Is the correction proper?
116 眼鏡をかけている	wear glasses
28 眼が見えなくなる	I went blind
126 目覚める (咳で)	wake up coughing
134 目覚める (夜中に)	wake up in the middle of the night
302 メジャーを当てて測る	measure it by using a tape measure
112 眼そのものは痛みませんか	Do you have any pain directly in or behind your eyes?
142 滅多にしないゴルフ	unusual golf swing
173 眼で追う (指先を)	Follow my finger with your eyes
30 眼にごみが入る	have a speck in my eye
112 眼の奥は痛みませんか	Do you have any pain directly in or behind your eyes?
70 眼の前が暗くなる	like swinging or fainting
118 眼の前で小さな虫が飛ぶ症状	symptom such as eye floaters
70 めまい (あなたの言う)	your dizziness
71 めまいを感じる	feel dizzy

101

278	目安にする(~リットル位を)	keep your urine output to ~ L
175	眼をそらさないで見る	focus on
187	眼を閉じて~する	do ~ with your eyes closed
189	眼を閉じて~する	close your eyes and do ~

も

268	も~もない(~)	There is no ~, nor ~
307	もう一枚(毛布を)	another blanket
311	申し訳ない(~して)	We apologize to have kept you waiting.
181	もう吸えないとなったら	When you can't get any more air in
173	もう少しあごを引く	tuck in your chin a little
307	毛布をかける	Would you like another blanket?
284	もし~でないなら	unless the TB organism is found
91	もしそうなら	If so
196	持ち上げる(両膝を腹の方に)	move them closer to your stomach
300	持ち上げる(シーツごと)	lift you together with the sheet
287	もちろん手術が(しかし)	but of course
301	持つ(腰を)	I'll grasp your lower back.
312	持って行く(窓口に)	take this folder to the receptionist
90	持っていたら(もし)	if you have them
217	持って来る(痰を)	bring the sputum in
297	持って来る(同意書を)	brings a consent form
316	持って来る(保険証を)	bring your health insurance card
132	元に戻る(数分で)	few minutes to recover
204	戻る(仰向けに)	Turn back over and lie on your back.
252	ものがある(~のように見える)	There are some structures which look like ~
8	物忘れ(母の)	my mother's forgetfulness
64	物を忘れる	forget things
29	も腫れている(喉)	My throat is swollen, too.
62	腿にあざができる	got a purplish bruise on my thigh
259	もやもやと見える	looks more whitish and wispy
288	模様をみる	see if that helps
168	盛り上がった	raised
21	モワーッとする(頭が)	My mind's foggy
222	問題が起きる	you will encounter more problems
246	問題がある(~に)	suggesting a problem with the heart valves

102

INDEX

104	問題はないですか(姿勢に)	Is there any problem with your posture?
	や	
224	夜間途中で目覚める	waking up often during the night
126	夜間も日中も	at night and during the day
80	焼き鳥	the grilled chicken
246	役立つ(〜に)	help with diagnosis
237	役に立つ運動	exercises that will help
310	役に立つ(浣腸液が)	the enema fluid will help
11	薬物治療(糖尿病の)	(or: medication) for diabetes
242	養う血管(〜領域を)	blood vessels feeding a stroke area
286	やすくする(痰を出し)	make it easier to bring up
133	休まずに歩く	without resting
271	休みだ(〜科が)	that department is not open
124	休む(学校を)	Were you frequently absent in elementary school
234	休める(身体を)	rest
236	休めること(身体を)	getting enough rest
223	痩せている	You look slim.
223	痩せる(どれ位)	How much weight did you lose
90	薬局の情報提供紙	package insert from the pharmacy
290	やってみましょう(〜かどうか)	Let's try first to break up the stone
238	止める(タバコを)	quit smoking
127	軟らかい(痰は)	Is it thin
286	軟らかくする(痰を)	thin the sputum
240	和らげる(痛みを)	a steroid to ease your pain
243	和げる薬(頭痛を)	one to ease the pain
	ゆ	
241	有効だ(体操も〜に)	exercise, may be helpful for 〜
15	歪んでいる(顔が)	My face feels a bit crooked.
140	指一本で示す	with one finger
189	指先で触る	with your fingertip
173	指先を追う	Follow my finger
213	指にはめる(センサーを)	wear that sensor on your finger
196	指を入れる(お尻に)	insert my finger into your anus
102	夢の中で金縛りになる	Have you ever dreamed about being paralyzed?
150	緩む(腹は)	have soft stools

103

70	揺れているような感じ	like swinging

よ

221	容器(そのための)	the container for that
219	容器に入れる	put the sputum in the container
295	要求する項目(～が)	the requirement by ~
295	用紙(会社が指定する)	the form specified by the company
295	用紙(当院の)	our form
47	陽性(便潜血検査が)	the stool blood test was positive
6	ようだ(～の)	My father seems alert but a bit confused.
9	ようだ(～の)	It seems that ~
241	ようだ(～の)	I suspect your headache is ~
246	ようだ(～の)	suggesting ~
48	ようだ(ぎっくり腰の)	like I strained it
53	ようだ(小石が残っている)	It feels like some sand or dirt is left inside.
14	ようだ(微熱がある)	I think I have
168	ようだ(水膨れの)	Does it look like blisters?
70	ような感じ(天井や壁が回る)	like the ceiling or walls are rotating
107	ような感じだ(痰になる)	I feel like
131	ような食べ物(チョコレートの)	food such as tomato or chocolate
135	ような日常生活動作(着替えの)	daily activities such as changing clothes
59	ようなもの(しみの)	a kind of brownish age spot
157	ようなもの(粘液の)	what looks like a sticky fluid
310	ように(役に立つ)	so that the enema fluid will help
161	ように感じる(尿が残っている)	feel like you still need to urinate
218	ようにする(奥から出す)	try to cough up the sputum
37	ように見える(～が膿んでいる)	It looks like it has pus
190	ように見える(～の)	It looks as if there's
241	ように見えない(～である)	It seems there's nothing wrong
252	ように見える(ウニのとげの)	look like sea urchin spines
252	ように見える(～が～である)	It looks like ~ are ~
301	ヨーイショ	Good.
64	よくある(高齢者では)	is common with age
119	よく出る(くしゃみが)	sneeze often
12	良くなる(たべると)	Eating sweet things makes me feel better.
274	良くなる(症状が)	get better
243	よくみられる(若い女性に)	is common among young women
249	よく見られる(良性の疾患に)	is common with benign diseases

INDEX

282	横から撮る	take x-rays from your back, side
189	横に出す (腕を)	Extend your arm to one side
46	横になると	when I lay down
170	横に引く (口元を)	pull your lips sideways
196	横向きに寝る	lie down on your side
307	汚れたシーツ	any mess
17	よだれが流れる	I drool from one side of my mouth.
50	寄って行く (歩くと右に)	move to the right when walking
134	夜中に目覚める	wake up in the middle of the night
311	呼ばれる (先に)	was called before me
299	呼びます (～が)	~ will call you
315	呼ぶ (番号順に)	We will call you in numeric order.
243	予防する薬 (頭痛を)	one to prevent
83	予防接種を受ける (インフルエンザの)	had a flu shot
295	予防接種	immunization shots
236	予防には (インフルエンザの)	In order to prevent flu
293	予約 (検査の)	appointments today for the next exam
308	予約が一杯だ (その日は)	that date is booked
313	予約制です (通常の診療は)	regular office visits are usually by appointment
313	予約無しの患者	walk-ins
312	予約日 (次の)	your next appointment
293	予約をする (二回分の)	make 2 appointments
294	予約をとる (来週月曜日に)	make an appointment for you for next Monday
141	より早く治まる	Does the pain stop sooner
126	夜も昼も	at night and during the day
269	拠れば (検査に)	According to today's microscopic examination
50	よろめく (歩くと)	stagger
150	弱い (腹は)	have a weak stomach
255	弱っている (心臓が)	You have some heart weakness
130	4分の1位	About 1/4 (a quarter)

ら

191	楽にする	relax your abdomen (or: stomach)
43	楽になる (こわばり感は)	The stiffness is better

241	ラジオ体操	radio exercise
248	らしくない(心筋梗塞)	It is not likely that
	り	
299	理学療法室	room for physiotherapy
299	理学療法士	physiotherapist
299	リハビリがある	you'll have a blood exam (x-ray exam, rehabilitation)
237	リハビリになる運動	exercises that will help
81	流行(インフルエンザの)	an outbreak of the flu
250	領域に(この白っぽい)	in this whitish area
240	良性の病気だ	This condition is benign
196	両膝を腹の方に持ち上げる	move them closer to your stomach
113	両耳で	in both ears
93	緑内障と言われた	had glaucoma
110	旅行に行く	go on a trip
235	旅行に行くにしても	may be going on a trip
	れ	
79	冷蔵庫で保管する	in a refrigerator
64	例をあげる(〜の)	Give me an example of ~
80	レストランで	in a restaurant
249	レベルでの(乳首の)	at the level of the nipple
143	レントゲンが引っかかる	An abnormal chest x-ray was found
268	レントゲン写真	x-ray image
299	レントゲン検査がある	you'll have a blood exam (x-ray exam
299	レントゲン室	x-ray room
299	レントゲン技師	x-ray technician
	ろ	
299	廊下の黄色い線	the yellow line in the corridor
138	労作時に	when you are exercising
256	労作時に	when exercising
248	労作性狭心症	angina on effort
250	肋骨と同じ位白い	is as white as ribs
16	呂律が回らない	can't speak distinctly
	わ	
19	わからない(味が)	food seems to lose its taste
38	腋の下に	in my armpit

INDEX

146	脇腹が痛む (左)	Did the right upper (lower, left) side of your stomach hurt?
249	輪切り像	the cross-section
83	ワクチン接種 (インフルエンザの)	a flu shot
289	分けて飲む (数回に)	several times per day
64	忘れた事 (お母さんが)	something that your mother has forgotten
317	渡す (処方箋を)	We will give you a prescription.
221	渡す (容器を)	I will give you the container
229	割には (写真の所見の)	The x-ray findings are of some concern, but
75	悪い物を食べる	ate some bad food
241	悪いものがあるように見えない (～に)	It seems there's nothing wrong in ~
265	悪いものを体の外に出す	let bad things leave the body
75	悪くなる (食べ物が)	it had gone bad
274	悪くなる (症状が)	get worse
290	悪さをしている (～が)	Your problem is due to ~

Phrase-book for care-givers

医師・看護師の英語フレーズブック

2014年6月20日　第1版第1刷 ©

著　　　者	佐藤　忍
	James P. Butler
発　行　人	尾島　茂
発　行　所	株式会社 カイ書林
	〒113-0021　東京都文京区本駒込4丁目26-6
	電話　03-5685-5802　FAX　03-5685-5805
	Eメール　generalist@kai-shorin.co.jp
	HPアドレス　http://kai-shorin.com
	ISBN　978-4-904865-15-6　C3047
	定価は裏表紙に表示
印 刷 製 本	モリモト印刷株式会社
	© Shinobu Satou

JCOPY ＜(社)出版者著作権管理機構 委託出版物＞

本書の無断複写は著作権法上での例外を除き禁じられています．複写される場合は，そのつど事前に，(社)出版者著作権管理機構 (電話 03-3513-6969, FAX 03-3513-6979, e-mail: info@jcopy.or.jp) の許諾を得てください．